The Sleep
Management Plan

The Sleep Management Plan

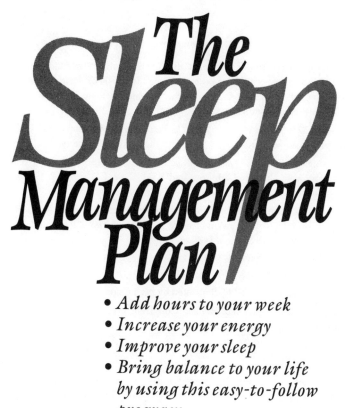

- *Add hours to your week*
- *Increase your energy*
- *Improve your sleep*
- *Bring balance to your life by using this easy-to-follow program*

Dale Hanson Bourke

Foreword by Wallace B. Mendelson, M.D.

▟ HarperSanFrancisco
A Division of HarperCollins*Publishers*

Grateful acknowledgment is made for permission to reprint the following:

The chart "Average Sleep Time of Mammals" appearing on page 19, and the Owl and Lark Questionnaire on pages 54–57, from *Wide Awake at 3:00 A.M.: By Choice or By Chance?* by Richard M. Coleman. Copyright © 1986 by Richard M. Coleman. Reprinted with permission of W. H. Freeman and Company.

The chart on page 22 from *Current Concepts™: The Sleep Disorders,* by Peter Hauri, Ph.D. Reprinted with permission of Peter Hauri, Ph.D. and the Upjohn Company.

The chart on pages 36–37 from *The Journal of Psychosomatic Research,* no. 11, titled "The Social Readjustment Scale," by T. H. Holmes and R. H. Rabe. Copyright © 1967 by Pergamon Press, Inc. Reprinted with permission of Pergamon Press, Inc.

The chart on page 40 from *The Hibernation Response,* by Peter Whybrow, M.D. and Robert Bahr. Copyright © 1988 by Peter Whybrow, M.D. and Robert Bahr. Reprinted with permission of Arbor House, a division of William Morrow & Co.

Cartoon on page 7 from "Calvin & Hobbs." Copyright © 1986 by Universal Press Syndicate. Reprinted with permission. All rights reserved.

Cartoon on page 43 from "Garfield." Reprinted by permission of UFS, Inc.

Cartoon on page 60 from "Calvin & Hobbs." Copyright © 1987 by Universal Press Syndicate. Reprinted with permission. All rights reserved.

Cartoon on page 121 from "Garfield." Reprinted by permission of UFS, Inc.

FIRST EDITION

Library of Congress Cataloging-in-Publication Data
Bourke, Dale Hanson.
    The sleep management plan / Dale Hanson Bourke—1st ed.
      p. cm.
    Contents: Includes bibliographical references.
    ISBN 0–06–250110–0
    ISBN 0–06–250113–5 (pbk.)
    1. Sleep—Health aspects.   I. Title.
RA786.B68 1990
613.7′9—dc20   89–45554
                                                        CIP

---

90   91   92   93   94 HAD 10 9 8 7 6 5 4 3 2 1

This edition is printed on acid-free paper that meets the American National Standards Institute Z39.48 Standard.

Contents

Acknowledgements   *vii*

Foreword by Wallace B. Mendelson, M.D.   *ix*

Introduction   *1*

Background

1. The 13-Month Year   5
2. Sleep 101   17
3. The Great Escape   33

The Sleep Management Plan

4. Step 1: Self-Assessment   47
5. Step 2: Motivation   63
6. Step 3: Organization   77
7. Step 4: Patterning   87
8. Step 5: Diet and Exercise   99
9. Step 6: Efficient Sleep   113
10. Questions and Answers   125

Appendixes

- Sleep Clinics   131
- Where to Find a Light Box   143
- Sunrise, Sunset Times for 2 Latitudes   144

Notes   *145*

Selected Bibliography   *147*

Acknowledgments

My curiosity about sleep might never have taken form in this book had it not been for the help of several doctors and other sleep professionals who generously offered encouragement, knowledge, and critiques. I am very grateful to the following people who were willing to help me: Bradford Kleinman, M.D.; Donald Bennett, M.D., Ph.D.; David Sack, M.D.; Michael Bonnet, M.D., Ph.D.; Peter Hauri, Ph.D.; William Dement, M.D., Ph.D.; and Wallace B. Mendelson, M.D.

I am also grateful to Jan Johnson and my friends at Harper San Francisco who caught the vision for this book and helped to shape it.

Thanks to the relatives, friends, and total strangers who were willing to share their personal experiences with me.

And to my family, who not only put up with my time at the computer, but also with all those bumps in the night as I conducted my own sleep experiments, I thank you and wish you sweet dreams.

Foreword

by Wallace B. Mendelson, M.D.

Sleep has been described by one well-known expert, Dr. Wilse Webb, as "the gentle tyrant." This phrase points to two important aspects of the need for sleep. On the one hand, it is imperative. It is a vital period of restoration that leads to healthy wakefulness during the day. In very extreme and unusual situations, in which animals are forcibly kept awake for long periods of time, or in which people have very rare degenerative diseases of the brain, long-term sleeplessness can lead to death. On the other hand, the tyrant is an understanding monarch who respects individual needs and is tolerant of some changes.

Ms. Bourke has written an exciting book, describing ways in which she has enriched her life by modifying her habits of sleeping, eating, exercising, and managing her time. It is a story of growth into a more active stance, in which she discovered that she was capable of being much more in charge of her own life than she had thought possible.

The theme that I see running throughout the book is an emphasis on individual differences. Thus, although there is indeed a basic need for a certain amount of sleep, there are great differences among individuals. Some persons fulfill their own needs, but stay in bed longer because they have heard that everybody needs a certain number of hours of sleep. The message Ms. Bourke shares with you is, "Listen to your own body; you can help determine for yourself how much sleep you need."

I think this is very sound advice. Ms. Bourke found that she did not need as many hours of sleep as she had thought. She combined her new schedule with new ways of thinking about her sleep, and new understanding of how her sleep relates to her daytime life. For instance, many people tend to think about their sleep in isolation, as if it is entirely separate from the rest of their lives. Ms. Bourke emphasizes how she discovered that sleep is influenced by her diet, exercise, how she deals with stress, and how she manages her time. Bringing all these things together led to a new, happier balance.

It should be emphasized that this is a book of self-improvement, not self-treatment. There are many medical reasons that could lead to a person feeling tired all the time. If you are tired all the time, I cannot emphasize too strongly that it is important to see your doctor, who will need to look for illnesses such as anemia, thyroid problems, and many other disorders. Similarly, this is not a guide for dealing with a long-term sleep disturbance. If you suffer from poor sleep or daytime sleepiness, it is important to be checked by a specialist in the many "hidden disorders of sleep" that can result in poor sleep. You alone will have to make that decision. Some of these disorders are described in chapter 2.

One good way to know that you are seeing a qualified specialist in such problems is to find a Sleep Disorder Center accredited by the Association of Sleep Disorder Centers (see the Appendix). One other word of caution: Although a small reduction in sleep usually has few medical consequences, common sense indicates that it can make you too sleepy in the daytime. It is important to listen to your own body, and not make yourself too sleepy. More important, you certainly would not want to drive or operate dangerous machinery, or otherwise put yourself in a position in which you could accidentally come into harm from being too sleepy.

Perhaps most important, remember that sleep is a part of your life. It is not some strange event that just happens to you. It is influenced by temperature and sunlight, your own personal physical and mental health, and to some extent reflects what has happened to you each day. Some of these factors are very much under your control. Just by addressing the topic you are already doing something useful—taking some time out from the many demands you must deal with and looking into doing something just for you. Try to learn more of what your own individual needs are. Ms. Bourke did this, and had a very happy personal experience of growth. I wish you a good journey on this same path.

Wallace B. Mendelson, M.D.
Director, Sleep Disorders Center
State University of New York at Stony Brook
Health Sciences Center

Introduction

"What type of book are you writing?" friends would ask when they heard I was spending my days in front of the computer.

After a conversation or two, I learned that all I had to say was, "It's about sleep." Almost everyone would respond with, "That's interesting. You know, I heard once . . ." or, "My favorite subject. If I don't get 8 hours I'm dead . . ." or, "I'm married to an insomniac."

Sleep, I have learned, is one of those very personal subjects that most of us are willing to talk about to a total stranger. After all, we're all experts on the subject. Each day we spend as much as one-third of our time personally experiencing its benefits. Besides our own experience, we have accumulated sayings and truisms that guide our beliefs on sleep. We know what we know—or do we?

When I began my personal investigation into sleep, I was adamant about my beliefs. I had 35 years of personal experience to back me up. Yet today I marvel at the lack of scientific and medical facts behind my assumptions. And I am amazed that I let my closed mind keep me from experiencing the rewards I now enjoy each day.

How has my life changed since I began my study of sleep?

- I feel better, day in and day out, than I can ever remember feeling before.
- I have more physical and mental energy.

- I am more optimistic and have fewer bouts with the blues.
- I have a more fulfilled family life because I have more time with my family and I am less anxious when I am with them.
- I feel better about myself because I have lost 10 pounds and am in better physical shape through regular exercise.
- I am generally more peaceful and serene and have a more meaningful spiritual life.
- I have developed new interests and am fascinated with areas I didn't know existed before.
- Stress is only an occasional visitor, not a regular inhabitant of my life.
- If I could sum up the change in my life over the past year, I would use one word: balance. I have a sense of balance in my life that simply did not exist before.

What does all this have to do with sleep? Nothing and everything. I have been able to achieve all these rewards *by sleeping only as much as I really need*. I actually sleep fewer hours each night and feel better physically, mentally, and spiritually.

> *I was no longer willing to give up*
> *one-third of my life without questioning*
> *the need for it or the benefits of it.*

If you are like most people, you may be saying, "Wait a minute. Don't tell me that I can actually feel *better* by sleeping less. I know how I feel. I'm exhausted. Crabby. I look terrible and I feel terrible. I've tried it and I know."

I wouldn't try to argue with you, because I was at exactly that point a year ago. But once I studied the medical facts, I felt I had to be open to changes in my behavior. I was no longer willing to give up one-third of my life without questioning the need for it or the benefits of it. So I tried a number of experiments, using myself as a guinea pig. Some were total failures. But finally I worked out a system that worked for me. By using it I reduced my nightly sleep from 8 hours to $6^1/2$ hours. I call this approach the sleep management plan.

Sleep reduction was my original goal. But after I was about halfway through the program, I found that the benefits I listed above were such strong incentives, that sleep reduction itself became a side issue. Sleeping only as much as I really needed offered me a way to achieve balance in my life. Sleep management began to take on a whole new meaning. I found that it allowed me to reduce my sleep, improve the sleep I did get, and *improve my waking hours.*

If you are picking up this book and wondering if it's worth the time to read it, take this simple quiz:

	YES	NO
Do I feel "stressed out" most days?	❏	❏
Do I wish I had more time to spend with friends and loved ones?	❏	❏
Do I fail to get the regular exercise I need to feel and look fit?	❏	❏
Do I miss time just for me—for hobbies, new interests, just relaxing?	❏	❏
Do I struggle with my self-image?	❏	❏
Do I live my family life on "fast forward"?	❏	❏
Do I end my day feeling that I've accomplished little and wonder where the day went?	❏	❏
Do I often feel tired?	❏	❏

If you answered yes to three or more of these questions, say yes to the sleep management plan. Try it for 2 weeks and experience some of the personal benefits yourself. Try it for 2 months and change your life. I did. And that's why this book is so important to me. In many ways it's my own story. But I believe it can easily be your story, too.

SLEEPFACT: Charles Dickens always slept with his head facing north so that his body would be in line with the earth's magnetic forces.

Chapter One

The 13-Month Year

Even where sleep is concerned, too much is a bad thing.
—Homer, *Odyssey*

It all began with a casual conversation. A business acquaintance and I were discussing our mutual love of tennis. I confessed that I just couldn't find time to play anymore. He said he played twice a week. I knew he held a demanding position in a growing organization, was active in civic affairs, and very involved with his family, so I asked the obvious question: "How do you find the time?" I am not being overly dramatic when I say that his answer changed my life.

"I get up around 5 A.M. and play before my family's awake," he said. Doing a quick calculation, I asked my follow-up question: "Then how much sleep do you get each night?"

He seemed a little embarrassed as he admitted that six hours was his normal amount of sleep. It didn't take me long to realize that this man had 2 more hours available to him each and every day than I did. While I was sleeping away he was already up, playing tennis, getting a head start on his work, doing whatever he wanted with his extra time. Each week he had 14 more hours than I did. Each month he had 60 more. Annually, the man was living an extra 700 hours while I was unconscious!

I had read every time-management book available. I faithfully carried my Filofax with me wherever I went. I made a daily to-do list. But it all seemed futile when I realized that this man lived a 13-month year. He had an extra month of waking hours available to him while I snoozed away.

The realization aroused my competitive nature. But it also made me see that all the things I longed for—time for myself, time for my family, time to just think—could be available to me if only I were lucky enough to sleep as little as my friend.

Luck was what I believed he had. After all, it didn't seem natural to sleep less than eight hours. He was probably doing terrible damage to his health, I reasoned. He might be taxing his heart unnecessarily. I was certainly doing the right thing by sleeping 8 hours each night—or was I?

My friend *looked* healthy. He seemed quite energetic and quick-witted, in fact. I, on the other hand, had been feeling increasingly sluggish and loved sleeping in on weekends whenever I had the opportunity. I assumed that the demands of work and the needs of 2 children were draining my energy. But what if I could find just an extra half hour in every day? Wouldn't that help ease the stress in my life and give me more energy?

An extra half hour in each day would give me 15 "bonus" hours each month and 182 hours each year.

It seemed like a catch-22. I didn't have enough time to get everything done, so I felt stressed. But the more stress I experienced, the more I wanted—even needed—sleep. In a way my response to sleep was the same response I had to food. The more weight I gained, the more I sought comfort from food.

A month after my conversation with my tennis-playing friend, I was having a cup of coffee with a man who not only ran a publishing company, but was the author of several books himself. Since it was evening, I was drinking my usual cup of decaf. He, on the other hand, ordered regular coffee and drank 2 cups. "Won't that keep you awake?" I asked.

"No problem," he said. "I usually stay up late and write. I've done most of my writing at all-night donut shops." I don't think I would have been more shocked if the man had confessed to some terrible crime. I'd known him for years. He'd taught me how to edit a magazine and we'd had dozens of philosophical discussions. But I never knew that he only slept so few hours each night. It seemed strange to think of this man sitting at the counter in a donut shop while most people were soundly sleeping. No wonder he accomplished so much!

The two conversations kept coming back to me. What if I didn't need as much sleep as I was getting? Was there a way to find time for tennis, for writing, for doing all those things I dreamed of? I decided it was worth taking time to explore the topic.

The Search Begins

What did I know about sleep when I began my search? Very little, really. My knowledge was similar to most people's—a combination of sayings, old wives' tales, my mother's wisdom, and what I thought was generally accepted medical advice:

- "You need your sleep."
- "Get a good night's sleep. You'll feel better in the morning."
- "Sleep on it."
- "Take 2 aspirin and call me in the morning."

I have had 2 children and survived months of irregular night-time feedings, so I knew that a person couldn't die from lack of sleep—even though you could feel so terrible you thought you might welcome death. But I also carried with me a sense that those all-nighters in college had taken their toll on my health. And no matter who was a guest on "The Tonight Show," I wasn't

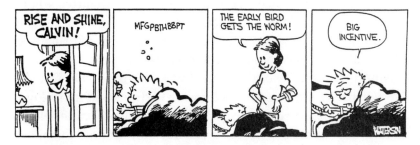

Much of what we "know" about sleep is based on folk wisdom.

going to ruin my health by staying up past midnight. I just *knew* I would fall apart the next day.

One day I went to see my doctor for a postnatal checkup, and I asked him what he knew about the medical needs for sleep. Having been awake for 24 hours himself delivering babies, he laughed. "Don't ask me. I'd love to find a way to survive on less," he said.

"But didn't you learn anything about sleep in medical school?" I asked.

"Just that you wouldn't get much sleep if you became a doctor," he said. "Actually, I think we had a lecture or two on sleep, but that's about all. If you're really interested, you should probably talk to a neurologist. Those are the guys who must know about sleep." He jotted down the name of a neurologist he knew and suggested that I call him.

I was becoming intrigued enough to make an appointment. "What's the problem?" the neurologist asked when I met him.

"It's not exactly a problem," I confessed. "I was wondering if I could get by on less sleep. It seemed like I might need a checkup or something before I tried to cut back."

"That's why you're here?" the man asked, not hiding his irritation. "I don't know anything about sleep. You need one of those sleep specialists," he said, sounding as if he were recommending I go to an astrologist. "This is not a medical problem. You're wasting my time and yours," he said, and ushered me out of the office.

Not a medical problem? I was beginning to feel as if there were more questions than answers—and I thought I had started where I should have, with the medical community. In frustration, I called the American Medical Association and asked for help in finding a doctor who had some knowledge of sleep.

After talking to several people, I was referred to Dr. Donald Bennett, director of the AMA's division of drugs and toxicology. He had been involved in a sleep education study a decade before, and my experience did not surprise him. He admitted that most

Sleep Myths

1. EVERYONE NEEDS 8 HOURS OF SLEEP PER NIGHT TO BE HEALTHY.

   FACT: Needs for sleep vary from person to person and by age. The need for sleep is both physical and psychological. People may need more sleep during times of stress. In other cultures sleep norms vary, with people often sleeping more in the winter months and less in summer. Most sleep specialists consider 6 to 9 hours per night as a "normal" amount of sleep.

2. THE AVERAGE DOCTOR KNOWS A GREAT DEAL ABOUT SLEEP.

   FACT: Most medical schools offer 2 or 3 lectures on sleep, mostly dealing with severe sleep dysfunctions.

   Most doctors are severely sleep deprived during training and while on call. Several studies have been done to see if this affects their work.

   The doctors who have studied sleep extensively are most likely to report that very little is really known about sleep. Doctors with little formal training in sleep are more likely to repeat conventional wisdom as medical fact.

3. WE CAN'T REALLY CONTROL OUR SLEEP PATTERNS.

   FACT: We can control our appetite for sleep just as we can control our appetite for food.

   Sleep patterns can be reestablished in approximately 3 weeks.

   Shift workers, pilots, physicians, and others routinely change their sleep patterns to accommodate work schedules and time changes.

4. IF WE FEEL TIRED, WE PROBABLY DIDN'T GET ENOUGH SLEEP.

   FACT: Being tired is often a symptom of the problems outlined in chapter 3, such as stress. Sleep reduction could actually help fight fatigue.

   We can learn to sleep more than we need just as we can learn to eat too much.

5. WE CAN'T CONTROL THE QUALITY OF OUR SLEEP.

   FACT: Poor sleeping patterns can often be managed and controlled.

   Many people who believe they suffer from insomnia get plenty of sleep; they just get poor-quality sleep.

doctors knew little about sleep. That's why the AMA had cooperated with the Department of Health and Human Services in developing a major program to educate doctors about sleep.[1] Unfortunately, funding for the program was cut before the materials could be widely distributed. But he was kind enough to send me a copy of the program, which included tapes, slides, and documents.

This was my first medical evidence that what I thought I knew about sleep was more fiction than fact. And what really surprised me was that the materials, aimed at educating practicing physicians, spent much time dispelling myths about sleep and sleep disorders.

Insomnia is a symptom; not a medical problem.

The material begins with a very elementary discussion of sleep patterns, and then moves into sleep disorders and one of the most common complaints physicians hear: "I just can't sleep." Surprisingly, this complaint is not viewed as serious. Dr. William Dement, a noted sleep authority from Stanford University, states that insomnia is a symptom, not a medical problem. And he goes on to say that unless the lack of sleep causes other medical problems, it probably does not require treatment at all.

Perhaps even more surprising is the fact that many people who claim they hardly sleep at all actually sleep quite a bit. When objectively measured in a sleep laboratory, people's perceptions of the amount of sleep they got versus the measured amount of sleep varied by as much as 4 to 6 hours a night.

Dr. Dement, in his advice to other doctors, states that people who claim to be insomniacs but who do not exhibit problems brought on by sleep loss fall into one of two categories: They either have inaccurate perceptions of how long they actually sleep, or are simply people *who do not need as much sleep as they think they need* but have somehow come to believe that their lack of sleep is abnormal.[2]

How Much Is Enough?

What started as a casual interest was becoming an obsession. I went to local and national libraries where I found volumes of materials on narcolepsy and other sleep disorders, but what seemed to be missing was information on *healthy* sleep patterns. Was it possible that 6 or 7 hours of sleep per night was just as healthy as 8? Was it possible that less sleep could even be better than more sleep?

I found a clue in an unlikely place. A small item in *USA Today* reported that Dr. David Sack, a psychiatrist from California, was

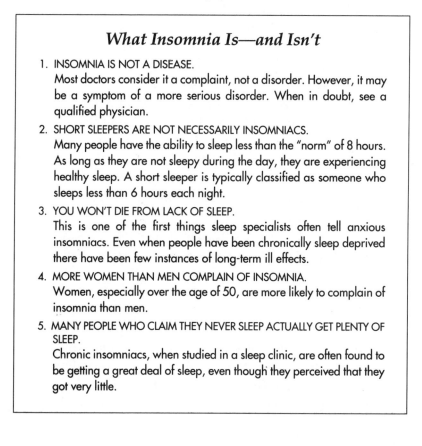

What Insomnia Is—and Isn't

1. INSOMNIA IS NOT A DISEASE.
   Most doctors consider it a complaint, not a disorder. However, it may be a symptom of a more serious disorder. When in doubt, see a qualified physician.

2. SHORT SLEEPERS ARE NOT NECESSARILY INSOMNIACS.
   Many people have the ability to sleep less than the "norm" of 8 hours. As long as they are not sleepy during the day, they are experiencing healthy sleep. A short sleeper is typically classified as someone who sleeps less than 6 hours each night.

3. YOU WON'T DIE FROM LACK OF SLEEP.
   This is one of the first things sleep specialists often tell anxious insomniacs. Even when people have been chronically sleep deprived there have been few instances of long-term ill effects.

4. MORE WOMEN THAN MEN COMPLAIN OF INSOMNIA.
   Women, especially over the age of 50, are more likely to complain of insomnia than men.

5. MANY PEOPLE WHO CLAIM THEY NEVER SLEEP ACTUALLY GET PLENTY OF SLEEP.
   Chronic insomniacs, when studied in a sleep clinic, are often found to be getting a great deal of sleep, even though they perceived that they got very little.

using a surprisingly simple short-term cure for some forms of depression: increased light and decreased sleep. His study showed that cutting sleep time in half "makes an immediate and very significant impact in treating depression."[3]

If less sleep was actually better for some people's mental health, didn't it follow that a "healthy" night's sleep might mean different things to different people?

When I interviewed Dr. Sack, I was surprised by his views of sleep. I expected him to give me very complex explanations of sleep theory. Instead, he said simply, "We do not know why we sleep."

The more I read, the more intrigued I became by the enormous gap between generally accepted sleep lore and what sleep experts had to say. Dr. Mangalore Pai, a British physician who established England's first sleep clinic, claimed that most people can survive—and thrive—on 5 to 6 hours of sleep per night. He considered sleeping longer to simply be "voluntary."[4]

His fellow countryman Dr. James Horne recently wrote a book entitled *Why We Sleep*. In it he asserts, "Despite 50 years of research, all we can conclude about the function of sleep is that it overcomes sleepiness, and that the only reliable finding from sleep deprivation experiments is that sleep loss makes us sleepy." Dr. Horne believes that the need for 7 to 8 hours of sleep each night is a myth and that most of us could cut back our sleep by 2 hours per night *without ill effects*.[5]

So why is there so much emphasis on insomnia? Lack of sleep as a problem is big business. I was astounded to read that 600 *tons* of sleep inducers are prescribed each year.[6] Many of these go to the elderly—especially women—who suffer from a wide range of disorders, with sleeplessness being one of the symptoms.

The growing concern over lack of sleep has also led to the development of sleep study departments in major hospitals and universities. And there are more than 100 sleep centers in the country accredited by the American Sleep Disorder Association (see the Appendix for a list). They are set up to work with people who suffer from such severe sleep-related problems as sleep apnea (cessation of breathing during sleep) to the more common complaints of fitful sleep.

It seemed that much of the emphasis on sleep in this country was to help deal with sleep problems. But I was beginning to believe that voluntary sleep reduction could offer significant benefits. In fact a study of a few years ago seemed to indicate that short sleepers in general are more energetic and outgoing, while longer sleepers tend to be more lethargic and depressive.[7]

Six hundred tons of sleep inducers are prescribed each year.

Some of history's greatest achievers were short sleepers. Thomas Edison considered sleep a waste of time. He reportedly slept an average of 4 hours per night. Benjamin Franklin wrote many of his sayings about time from personal experience. He slept as little as possible. Winston Churchill was famous for sleeping only a few hours at night and then taking a quick nap or two during the day. Napoleon slept only 3 or 4 hours each night.

Despite the regular reports of Ronald Reagan's love of sleep, most recent presidents have slept far less. Lyndon Johnson and Jimmy Carter were notoriously short sleepers while in office, averaging 5 hours sleep each. A recent article on President Bush reported that he and Barbara awaken every morning at 5 A.M. Considering the many social obligations they have in the evening, it seems reasonable to surmise that their average bedtime is well after 10 P.M.

Other short sleepers include Barbara Walters, Donald Trump, Ed McMahon, Bryant Gumble, Cloris Leachman, and George Plimpton. All these people are famous achievers. But short sleepers come in all shapes, sizes, and backgrounds. I began asking different people I knew about their average amount of sleep and found a surprising number of people I knew slept as little as 6 hours per night. Of course, 7 to 8 was the average for most people I asked; but people who slept less than that often

---

Contemporary and Historic Short Sleepers

Isaac Asimov	Thomas Edison	Ed McMahon
Napoleon Bonaparte	Benjamin Franklin	Deborah Norville
George Bush	Bryant Gumble	Danielle Steel
Jimmy Carter	Lyndon Johnson	Barbara Walters
Charles Dickens	Edward Koch	

---

confessed that their spouses thought something was wrong with them, or that they didn't tell people how little they slept because they felt like oddballs.

One doctor I know, who is from South America, told me simply, "Americans sleep too much." He explained that when he was in medical school he learned that the average person who lives to be 75 has slept away 25 years of life. That was all the incentive he needed to cut back his sleep to only 5 hours each night. "This way I get a few extra years," he told me good-naturedly.

Another man confessed that the fact that he slept only 5 hours each night was a major source of irritation to his wife, who thought it was unhealthy. When I told him about some of the medical research I had uncovered he was relieved and later reported that his wife had decided to try to cut back on her sleep, too.

A 50-year-old woman told me she was forced to cut back her sleeping hours when she had 4 children under the age of 5. Realizing that she didn't feel so bad after all, she continued to sleep less than 6 hours a night, even after the children were grown. "Now I use the time for me!" she reported.

A man I met on an airplane told me he'd learned to sleep less while sailing solo for weeks. Once he quit sailing he never went back to sleeping more than 5 hours at a time.

One minister I met mentioned that awakening early to spend time in prayer and Bible study had made a major difference in his spiritual life. "And when my spiritual life is in good shape I don't *need* as much sleep," he said.

Yes, But . . .

At this point in my research, I asked the obvious question— and you may be asking it too: "If I don't really *need* 8 hours of sleep, why do I feel so lousy without it?"

Human beings are remarkably adaptable creatures, and our response to sleep seems to be one indication of our flexibility. Just as some of us can eat 1,500 calories a day while others consume 3,000 to 4,000 calories, each of us has a different disposition, metabolic rate, and life-style that may contribute to what we feel is our need for sleep.

If you really wanted to, you could probably sleep an *additional* 2 hours each night without major side effects. But you could also possibly sleep 2 hours less than you currently do. The fact is we don't like change and once we are accustomed to 3,000 calories or 8 hours of sleep, our bodies resist new patterns.

The body's mechanism for controlling sleep needs is remarkably simple, not unlike a thermostat.

Sleep reduction, I have found through personal experience, is not accomplished quickly or without commitment. But you can teach your body to adapt to less sleep in approximately the same way you train yourself to eat less when you diet. The first few days can be uncomfortable as you try to unlearn the habits of a lifetime. But it is easier to stay on a diet after a week or two as your body adapts to fewer calories. The same is true of sleep reduction.

The body's mechanism for controlling sleep needs is not unlike a thermostat. It uses physical and mental information to decide when to signal the onset of sleep and when to send out a "rise and shine" impulse. But this "sleepostat" can be adjusted and reset.

I am a living example of a person who, just over a year ago, thought that 8 hours of sleep a night was a minimum requirement for feeling decent and having some degree of mental stability. I was absolutely sure that to sleep less would leave me feeling lousy. It did, for the first few days. But today I sleep an average of 6½ hours a night and have never felt better in my life. I rarely drink coffee or colas (5 cups of coffee and 2 cola drinks were my norm when I slept 8 hours) and I have more energy than I had when I was 18. I am not a particularly self-disciplined person, and I juggle the demands of a household and a business.

The methods that worked for me can work for anyone. So if you think that maybe, just maybe, you could use an extra hour or two each day for the rest of your life, read on.

SLEEPFACT: John Wesley's bedtime ritual included taking a cold bath and going to bed without drying himself off.

Chapter Two

Sleep 101

Sleep is the most moronic fraternity in the world, with
the heaviest dues and the crudest rituals.
—Vladimir Nabokov

Surely I was missing something. It seemed amazing to me that
I had willingly given up one-third of my life without any real
basis. How had so many people come to believe that it was
"right" to sleep 8 hours?

I decided to study everything I could about sleep. I enrolled
myself in Sleep 101 (a self-study course) and began to read
medical journals, newspaper articles, and books by the stack. I
didn't have to read very much to discover that most experts
agreed on the basic facts of sleep.

Why We Sleep

Aristotle thought he had it figured out nearly 2,000 years ago.
We fall asleep, he concluded, because of rising vapors from our
stomach. It was all a function of the digestive system, in his
opinion, and that was why we often grow tired after eating.

As absurd as his theory may seem, we have made surprisingly
little progress in finding a more definitive explanation. At one
point experts believed that sleep was caused by "congestion of
the brain" by excessive blood. This is probably why we use
pillows, since elevating the head was thought to reduce this
congestion. Another theory purported that sleep was in fact
caused by the *absence* of blood in the head.[1] (Perhaps the pillow-
makers' lobby effectively squelched this idea.)

Scientists know why we eat, the function of water and fluids,
and the importance of exercise. Yet why we sleep still baffles

some of the best brains in the world. "When you start to ask the question, 'What is the function of sleep?' it's the same as asking 'What is the function of wakefulness?'" says Dr. Anthony Kales, director of the Sleep Research and Treatment Center at Pennsylvania State University's Milton S. Hershey Medical Center. "I don't know the function of being awake any more than I know the function of being asleep."[2]

In traditional cultures sleep is often viewed as an aid to survival; a time to keep out of the path of enemies. In contemporary Western culture, some behaviorists believe that sleep is a way of keeping us occupied so we don't grow bored, or of simply escaping the stress of daily life.[3]

In many cultures sleeping hours vary dramatically by season.

Although most people imagine that there is something almost sacred about sleeping 8 hours a night, this norm was established relatively recently in our society, mostly in response to the industrial revolution and industry's need for regulation. When we were primarily an agricultural society, we arose and went to bed with the sun.

This is still true in many cultures today, which means that sleeping hours vary dramatically by the season. In some parts of the world people sleep up to 12 hours in the winter months and half that in the summer. Scandinavian countries, though industrialized, still have widely varying patterns of sleep depending on the amount of sunlight available.[4]

An anthropologist friend of mine, who lived with the Masai tribe in Africa for a year, observed that the men slept only 3 to 4 hours each night and the women slightly longer. Others have studied the Temiar people of Malaysia and found that 6 hours of sleep is their norm.[5] Observing these differences among peoples of the world has convinced many scientists that the amount of sleep we consider normal is primarily a matter of personal and societal conditioning.

Dr. Peter Hauri, director of the Mayo Clinic's Insomnia Program, sums it up this way in his book *No More Sleepless Nights*:

> We don't expect everybody in the world to wear the same size shoes, but somehow people think that we should all sleep the same length of time.
>
> The amount of sleep that people need varies tremendously. There is no "normal" amount.[6]

Dr. Hauri goes on to quote figures from the National Health Center for Statistics, which state that in the United States 2 people out of 10 sleep less than 6 hours each night.

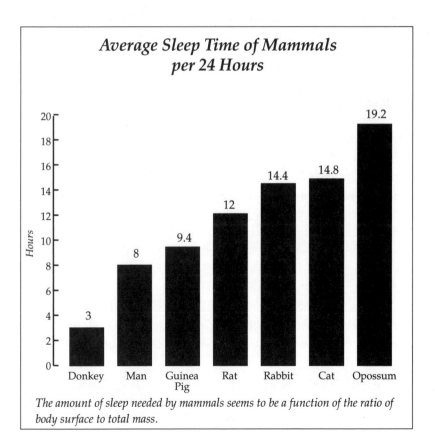

The amount of sleep needed by mammals seems to be a function of the ratio of body surface to total mass.

Theories of Sleep

Basically, there are two major theories of sleep: the restorative theory and the adaptive theory. The restorative theory is the older, and may account for the common "wisdom" that sleep is critical for good health.

The restorative theory was developed when doctors thought our bodies simply "shut down" during sleep, causing a mini-hibernation during every 24-hour period. Ancient superstition held that during sleep we came close to death, and an often-used bedtime prayer is based on this assumption: "Now I lay me down to sleep, I pray the Lord my soul to keep. If I should die before I wake, I pray the Lord my soul to take."

Neither the mind nor the body shuts down during sleep.

We know now that neither the mind nor the body shuts down during sleep. Both are actually quite active. Human cells die and are replaced constantly during the day and night, but there is some evidence to suggest that there is a greater activity level during sleeping hours.

Growth hormones are also especially active during sleeping hours. Scientists have found that this is especially true in children and adolescents.[7] Other hormones seem to be more concentrated during sleep.

Some restorative theories have come under attack, especially in recent years, as scientists observe sleep in a more controlled environment and can make a better connection between cause and effect.

The adaptive theory says basically that sleep is learned behavior, something that has been passed down through the ages. According to Wilse Webb, a proponent of this theory:

> Sleep developed, in the particular forms and patterns it took in each species, as a behavior that increased the likelihood of that species' survival. The particular survival value associated with sleeping—that of reducing behavioral activity—was to

protect the animal (including man) from dangerous or ineffi-
cient activities, both his own and others', particularly in
reaction to foraging or food gathering. Sleep, then, evolved in
each species as a form of "nonbehavior" when not responding
in the environment would increase survival chances. [8]

If we have, in fact, learned to sleep, could it be that we might
unlearn this behavior, especially now that electricity gives us the
ability to control the light and temperature 24 hours a day?

Dr. Gordon G. Globus of the University of California at Irvine
says, "Because a number of factors such as less physical work to
accomplish and better nutrition, our bodies may not need any-
where near as much sleep as we actually obtain, but our brains
continue to impose this evolutionary anachronism on us."[9]

And Dr. Pai believes that we may see a general tendency for
people to sleep less in the future. "It is part of man's evolutionary
process that he should sleep less and less as he discovers more
reasons for staying awake." [10]

Although no one really knows why we sleep, in the past few
years scientists have discovered a great deal about the *patterns* of
our sleep.

Sleep Patterns

Doctors and researchers have studied sleep patterns extensively and can document the typical pattern during an average
night's sleep. Sleep is roughly divided into REM (rapid eye
movement) and non-REM periods.[11]

Many people believe that dreaming occurs during the deepest
moments of sleep, but actually we dream during REM sleep,
which some researchers call one of the "shallowest" stages of
sleep. We are easily awakened by noises during REM sleep. That
is why we often have the sense of awakening in the middle of a
dream. The fact is that most of us move from REM sleep into
wakefulness, and the ringing of the alarm clock or the stirring of
our spouse may pull us out of a dream and into consciousness
rather abruptly.

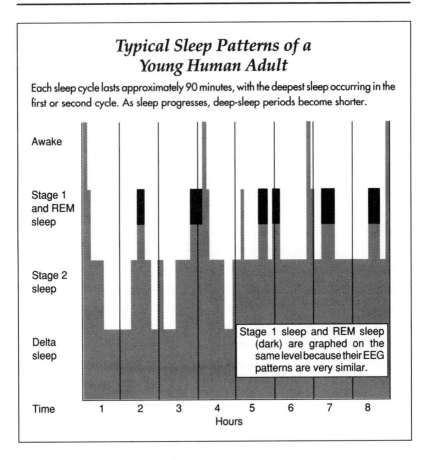

Typical Sleep Patterns of a Young Human Adult

Each sleep cycle lasts approximately 90 minutes, with the deepest sleep occurring in the first or second cycle. As sleep progresses, deep-sleep periods become shorter.

Awake

Stage 1
and REM
sleep

Stage 2
sleep

Delta
sleep

Stage 1 sleep and REM sleep (dark) are graphed on the same level because their EEG patterns are very similar.

Time   1   2   3   4   5   6   7   8
                        Hours

Non-REM sleep is divided into 4 stages. Stage 4, the deepest sleep, occurs most often in the earliest hours of a night's sleep. Typically, we fall into non-REM sleep rapidly. After about half an hour we may move back into lighter sleep, experiencing our first REM sleep an average of 90 minutes after we first lose consciousness. A short period of REM sleep is followed by a more gradual descent into what is most often our last Stage 4 sleep of the night. *By the time we have been asleep for less than 3 hours, most of us will have completed our deepest sleep of the night.*

Between our third and fourth hour of sleep we will repeat the descent. But this time we will go only into Stage 3 sleep before gradually returning to what will be the longest REM period of the night. Much of the time between our fourth and fifth hour of sleep is given to REM sleep, and possibly dreaming. Because dreaming is considered so psychologically beneficial, this period of sleep must be viewed as valuable, even though it is not deep sleep, which is believed to have the most physically restorative effects. But at the end of our fifth hour of sleep, we will probably not sleep any more deeply than Stage 2. We may experience another REM period just before we awaken. Despite the fact that we may complain as the alarm goes off, "But I was sleeping so deeply," the fact is that we spend the time after our fifth hour of sleep very close to wakefulness.

Dr. Horne considers this period of sleep "superflous."[12] Although there may be some evidence to support our physical need for sleep in Stages 3 and 4, and our psychological need for REM sleep and dreaming, the last 2 to 3 hours of the 8-hour-a-night sleeper are called "optional" by Dr. Horne.

We are easily awakened by noises during REM sleep.

This pattern is predictable in most people, but studying it helps doctors understand more about serious sleep disorders. Sleep apnea, for example, is characterized by loud snoring. People with this condition literally stop breathing while asleep. The "snoring" is actually the person gasping for breath and, in the process, being awakened hundreds of times during the night. The regular sleep cycle never has a chance to begin.

Some people never descend into the deepest stages of sleep. Ironically, sleeping pills, which are effective in bringing on sleep, seem to inhibit deep sleep. A person who has taken sleeping pills may fall asleep quickly and even sleep for 10 hours, but the sleep may be of poor quality, leaving the person exhausted.

Alcohol is another enemy of Stage 3 and 4 sleep. Drinking too much may help a person feel sleepy, but chances are that sleep will be of poor quality. Even a single drink before bedtime can be detrimental to the important first hours of sleep, and a person may never experience the deepest sleep, even after long hours of sleep.

The Circadian Clock

We are all vaguely aware of our internal biological clock that signals hunger even when we are not watching the time or causes us to grow tired as our normal bedtime nears. Even without environmental cues, our clocks seem to try to help us maintain a regular rhythm to our life. Our circadian clock is simply our daily cycle. Although we have learned to operate on a 24-hour day, left completely free of restrictions most of us would actually function on a 25-hour day. In fact, people without any sense of day and night tend to "free run," often staying awake for 20 hours or more, then sleeping for 10 to 12 hours. Free running is observing a cycle of one's own rather than a cycle imposed by outside influences. (This concept was not understood during the 1800s when world time was first standardized.)[13] Other mammals operate on different circadian cycles.

> *People without any sense of day and night tend to "free run," often staying awake for 20 hours or more, then sleeping for 10 to 12 hours.*

Scientists have never actually located "the clock" in anyone's body, but they can determine how the clock is functioning by measuring body temperature and certain hormone outputs. In fact, we can chart our own daily cycle by using a basal thermometer and noting temperatures at each hour during the day (and, if you are so inclined, during the night).

One of the most fascinating aspects of the circadian rhythm is how body temperature relates to sleep. Temperature begins to fall a few hours before one's normal bedtime and begins to rise again just before waking. In many ways the circadian clock is the body's "sleepostat," which more than any other cue signals bedtime.

every fall and spring as we change our schedules to accommodate daylight savings time. In addition, we change our clocks
more drastically when we travel across time zones. Shift workers
must dramatically reset their circadian cycles and often experience great difficulty in functioning for the first week after their
schedule has been inverted. (A fascinating book on this topic is
Richard M. Coleman's *Wide Awake at 3:00 A.M.*)

But we can reset our sleepostat in as little as 3 to 10 days and
begin to function normally. Our body simply learns from the
pattern set the day and night before. That is why we have so
much difficulty awakening on Monday morning after sleeping in
on Saturday and Sunday. Our circadian clock has begun to shift
to a later time and is beginning to stabilize our routine.

Sleep Loss

What happens when we don't sleep? We all know how we feel:
irritable, unresponsive, "draggy." Sometimes we experience
headaches, burning eyes, and an upset stomach. But for all the
symptoms, surprisingly little harm comes to us when we get little
or no sleep.

I had come to believe all sorts of myths about sleep loss,
perhaps extrapolating how bad I could feel after a short night to
what a person must experience after severe sleep loss. A friend's
father had a heart attack, which was blamed on the fact that he
was a very short sleeper. I had heard that one would hallucinate
after a few days of sleep loss and that it was possible to actually
cause a shutdown of an entire body system if you went without
sleep. After searching through medical journals, however, I am
convinced that this was all from the body of knowledge that says
chicken soup can cure a cold and you can get warts from toads.

Says sleep expert Dr. Wallace Mendelson:

> The classic tool in biology for determining the function of
> some process is to deprive the body of that process and see
> what happens. If, for instance, you want to find out how a
> pancreas works, one classical method is to remove it from an

pancreas works, one classical method is to remove it from an animal and observe the results.

But when that technique is applied to sleep, it doesn't work. It's hard to find a clear physiological deficit in sleep deprivation. If you deprive someone of sleep for 200 to 250 hours, you can get some psychotic symptoms. Short of that extreme kind of deprivation, however, you see a very sleepy person, but it's almost impossible to point to clear deficits in specific processes.[14]

Early experiments in sleep deprivation used animals, and did show significant problems with their ability to adapt. One doctor I know, a general practitioner, said he thought loss of sleep was bad because he remembered the "famous puppy experiment." In this experiment puppies forced to go without sleep for long periods actually died, although now scientists dispute the findings because of the way the experiment was carried out and the methods for analysis.[15]

> *There is simply no medical evidence*
> *that too little sleep—either short- or long-term—*
> *causes lasting problems.*

Today doctors know that heat loss in small mammals is a major problem of sleep deprivation, something that larger mammals have less trouble dealing with because of a lower surface area ratio. And with sophisticated sleep labs and the ability to use EEGs, researchers are better able to study humans.

Studies on the effects of sleep deprivation in humans go on regularly, often funded by the U.S. military. At first I was surprised to find so much research coming out of Walter Reed Army Hospital and to discover researchers such as Dr. Michael Bonnet carrying on studies at the Veterans Hospital in Long Beach, California. But then he explained: "We need to know whether we can put troops on a transport plane, fly them overseas, and still expect them to be able to fight a battle without sleeping for 36 hours."

If the thought of a sleep-deprived army fighting a major battle frightens you, remember that most medical interns routinely work 36-hour shifts. Although recent investigations have focused on the mistakes made by sleep-deprived doctors, scientific studies show that skillful performance of intricate tasks is just as possible by a well-rested person as by a person who hasn't slept for as much as 48 hours.[16]

Says Dr. Ernest Hartmann, "There are few clearly demonstrated chemical-physiological changes produced by sleep deprivation." [17]

In 1965 Randy Gardner, observed by Stanford's Dr. Dement, set an official record by going 11 days without sleep. Gardner experienced few serious physical or mental problems, although he became irritable, slurred his speech, had blurred vision, and some memory loss. Yet on the last night of his ordeal he played pinball games by the hour and beat the well-rested doctor.

After the 11 days Randy slept for nearly 15 hours and seemed fully recovered.[18] In fact, the ability to fully recover after only sleeping for a fraction of the hours lost is another reason scientists believe that sleep loss is not truly harmful. Whether a person has lost a single night's sleep or several, approximately 25 percent of the lost sleep is all that is needed to "catch up."[19]

Approximately 25 percent of the lost sleep is all that is needed to "catch up."

Dr. Horne theorizes that some of the side effects of sleep loss are due to "cerebral impairment." But he emphasizes that this cerebral impairment is not to be viewed as brain damage, but a reversible state, analogous to the impairment and recovery of muscle after exercise. [20]

When doctors discovered that sleep deprivation could actually break a cycle of depression, they may have not only helped depressives, but also contributed to breaking the cycle of mythology that surrounds sleep loss. Sleep loss may not hurt; in fact, it might even help certain people.

"But I heard you would go crazy if you didn't dream," a friend said with great confidence. Experiments have been done to interrupt only REM sleep, theoretically disturbing sleep only during the times when dreams take place. Subjects did grow irritable, but none went crazy. Another myth debunked.

What Is Insomnia?

"Don't tell my husband about your book," one woman urged. "He's already an insomniac. He'll probably get worse." The woman was echoing another myth—that anyone who doesn't sleep the "normal" 7 to 8 hours per night is an insomniac.

Insomnia is one of the most often heard complaints by doctors—and one of the complaints taken least seriously. In fact Dr. Richard Podell wrote *Doctor, Why Am I So Tired?* because he often felt his colleagues too quickly dismissed people who were tired.[21] But being tired and not getting enough sleep are not necessarily the same thing.

Very simply, the word insomnia is derived from the Latin root that means "without sleep." Dozens of books have been written on the topic, and typically they concentrate on "getting to the root of insomnia." This is simply another way of saying that insomnia, in itself, is not a disease. The inability to sleep may or may not be a problem.

Being tired and not getting enough sleep are not necessarily the same thing.

"I generally measure the amount of sleep a person needs in terms of daytime alertness," says Dr. Donald Sweeney in *Overcoming Insomnia*. "My formula is simple: *If you go through the day wide awake, alert, and energetic, then you are getting enough sleep.*"[22]

As we have already seen, different cultures have different norms for sleep. An American insomniac would be considered an excessive sleeper by the Temiars. And the amount of sleep

Drugs that Contain Caffeine

MEDICINE	MILLIGRAMS OF CAFFEINE PER DOSE
Dexatrim	200
Vivarin	200
Cafergot	100
Migralam	100
No-Doz	100
Excedrin	65
Pre-Mens	65
Migral	50
Fiorinal	40
Anacin	30
Bromo-Seltzer	30
Cope	30
Vanquish	30

needed by individuals varies dramatically, although we can assume that many people succumb to some societal pressures and aim for the 8-hour norm.

All of us go through periods of our lives when stress, environment, or other factors keep us from sleeping. This is transient insomnia, sleeplessness that will pass when the circumstances change. Even if we do experience difficulty in functioning well the next day, it's helpful to remember that no serious harm is being done, and there is no reason to believe that transient insomnia will develop into chronic insomnia.

Chronic insomnia is often experienced by individuals who are having other physical problems or are dealing with difficult emotional or psychological situations. Some people can't sleep because of pain. Others can't sleep because a drug given to them to treat one problem is causing other disruptions.

Malsomnia is taken from the French word for "bad sleep," and simply means that a person does not sleep well. The malsomniac may sleep 8 or more hours per night but never feel rested. There can be many reasons for this, including alcohol, drugs, environmental problems, stress, or sleeping disorders.

Hypersomnia is excessive sleeping. Some hypersomniacs are also malsomniacs. Others have simply grown accustomed to a longer time in bed. Still others suffer from serious diseases—perhaps undiagnosed—that sap their energy, such as cancer.

Specialists agree that the number of hours we sleep each night is not nearly as important as the way we feel during our waking hours. And no matter how many hours of sleep we get, feeling tired during the day can be a symptom of a serious mental or physical problem. Telling yourself, "I just need to get more sleep," is not dealing with the underlying problem. Neither is taking a sleeping pill. If you feel tired, review the possible reasons in the next chapter, or read Dr. Podell's book.[23] And then *see a doctor* who takes your concerns seriously.

Although you probably won't die from lack of sleep, you can cause yourself serious harm by not dealing with the condition that causes your lack of sleep. Conversely, if you only sleep a few hours a night but feel fine during the day, relax and enjoy your naturally low need for sleep. You are not an insomniac. You are simply more fortunate than many of us who have been conditioned to believe that 8 hours of sleep ranks with apple pie and motherhood as great American virtues. According to Dr. Mendelson, "Questions such as 'How much sleep should I get?' cannot be answered by referring to tables, as in looking up an ideal body weight for a given height. Each person seems to have his or her own requirement for sleep."[24]

Sleep Disorders

My growing knowledge of sleep did two things for me. First, it took away my fear of sleep and the control it had over me. I no longer worried about getting a good night's sleep. If I wasn't able to get much sleep one night, I reminded myself that it was entirely possible for me to function well the next day and that only slightly more sleep the following night would "catch me up."

But I also developed a healthy respect for sleep—especially as I read more about sleep disorders, a relatively new field of study in medicine. Serious sleep disorders are only now being understood and taken seriously.

For example, snoring was considered nothing more than an annoying habit by most doctors, who prescribed nose drops for the problem until only a few years ago. Now it is understood that snoring may actually be a sign of sleep apnea, which simply means that a person stops breathing during sleep. Some doctors believe that sleep apnea is the true cause of Sudden Infant Death Syndrome (SIDS).

According to the AMA as many as 1 in 10 Americans may have seriously disturbed breathing during sleep.[25] Sleep apnea is typically characterized by loud and continuous snoring. The person with sleep apnea gets significantly less oxygen into the bloodstream, which may cause problems with the heart. In some cases the heart actually stops beating altogether for a moment. The person may also have periods of high blood pressure during sleep, which eventually continues into the waking hours.

According to the AMA, 1 in 10 Americans may have seriously disturbed breathing during sleep.

Sleep apnea occurs most often in those who are overweight and seems to be more prevalent in people over the age of 50. Naturally, a person who suffers from sleep apnea is tired during the day, because the previous night's sleep has been disturbed hundreds of times.

Cures for sleep apnea range from gently forcing air down the throat to prescribing a drug. Surgery is performed to correct a severe obstruction. Treating the problem is important, however, since doctors theorize that many heart attacks and strokes that occur during sleep are actually a result of this condition.

Narcolepsy is another serious sleep disorder that is character-ized by the inability of a person to stay awake—even at the most inappropriate moments. Although most of us have found our-selves dozing during a soothing concert, a boring lecture, or a long sermon, narcoleptics doze off regularly and may even fall asleep behind the wheel of their cars. Some narcoleptics are able to hide their symptoms well, but may suffer from hallucinations during the day. These episodes may actually be dreams or nightmares. Cataplexy, or the sudden loss of muscle control brought on by an emotional reaction, is also a common problem of narcoleptics.

Narcoleptics may get 8 hours or more of sleep at night, but still suffer from excessive daytime sleepiness. And with the additional symptoms of hallucinations and muscle "jerks" (the involuntary attempts by the body to keep the person awake), a person with narcolepsy may be diagnosed as having mental problems.

It is now known that narcolepsy is a disorder of the central nervous system and can often be treated with drugs. But many doctors still do not understand this disorder and misdiagnose it. Mild cases cause people to be labeled "lazy."

Narcolepsy is a very serious sleep disorder and one that has implications for every aspect of life. If you suspect you suffer from narcolepsy, it is important to see a sleep specialist who can help diagnose and treat this disorder.

Other sleep disorders include sleepwalking, regular leg movements during sleep, and sleep talking. If you suffer from any of these symptoms, see your doctor. Even if the symptoms aren't troublesome to you, they may indicate a more serious problem. If you do not feel that the doctor is taking your concerns seriously, ask to be referred to a sleep specialist. (See the Appendix for a directory of certified sleep centers.)

SLEEPFACT: In most people rapid-eye-movement sleep means that eyes move back and forth. But some pygmies have up-and-down eye movement during sleep—theoretically because they spend so much of their waking time looking up.

Chapter Three

The Great Escape

Early to bed and early to rise makes a man healthy,
wealthy, and wise.
—Benjamin Franklin

One of my favorite cartoons of all time has been tacked to my bulletin board for years. In it Snoopy is reminded that it is the first day of February. "What happened to July?" he exclaims. He bemoans the many things he has to do, places he wants to go, and things he wants to see. In the final frame we see him asleep on the roof of his doghouse. How I identify with this approach to life! When things seem most overwhelming sleep becomes a great escape from the pressures of daily living.

Some people, unable to cope with daily pressures, turn to alcohol or drugs. But for many of us sleep represents a socially acceptable respite from stresses or responsibilities. It gives us a chance to regroup, to ease the tension, to clear our minds. When we say, "I'm going to sleep on it," we sometimes mean, "I want to escape from the pressure of this decision." And, in fact, we sometimes do awaken to a new day with an accompanying fresh outlook. The hours of escape have eased the pressure and cleared our minds so that we are more able to make a tough decision or resolve a dilemma.

A Balanced View of Sleep

There is nothing wrong with using sleep as an escape. It is certainly a healthier physical and mental alternative than drugs, alcohol, or other substances. What *is* wrong is not recognizing that we are choosing to sleep and that the act is something we control.

I was absolutely amazed to discover that sleep is not inherently good. We are not necessarily improving our health, well-being, or performance by getting more sleep.

But neither is sleep bad. I have a friend who considers sleep "a total waste of time." He sometimes goes for days with little or no sleep. It seems clear that his view isn't totally balanced either.

A more balanced view of sleep would be similar to the way we view food. We need to eat every day and we have a wide range of foods from which to choose. Yet most of us eat too much of the wrong kinds of food. We have control of our diets to a great degree, but we sometimes choose the calorie-laden chocolate cake or the greasy potato chips. If we make these choices too often, we gain weight and have to deal with accompanying problems of poor self-image and possible health complications. Given the clear relationships between our behavior and the results, why do we choose to eat that piece of chocolate cake? The simple answer is that it tastes good. And sometimes the soothing nature of a gooey dessert may be more important to our state of mind than to the success of our diet.

> ### *We are not necessarily improving our health, well-being, or performance by getting more sleep.*

Inherently there is nothing wrong with food. If we eat too little we become too thin. If we eat too much we gain weight. We have a wide range of choice in terms of quantity of foods and types of foods. Most of us recognize that it is our choices that are right or wrong, not food itself.

So it is with sleep. We can get more than we need without side effects. And the desire to sleep is strong: "Next to sex and hunger, the urge to sleep is nature's most powerful drive," says Dr. Dement.[1]

Why Do I Feel Tired?

You may agree that sleep itself is neither good nor bad, but few people would find feeling tired to be any less than annoying, frustrating, and uncomfortable. No one *likes* to feel tired. And for years we have been taught that if you feel tired you haven't had enough sleep. Therefore sleep is considered a cure for one of the most common complaints of modern men and women.

Sometimes fatigue is a cry for help.

The fact is that people who sleep *too much* complain of the same symptoms as insomniacs: sluggishness, irritability, difficulty concentrating, and so on. And those of us who occasionally or regularly complain of the same symptoms may be neither insomniacs nor hypersomniacs. We may simply have other reasons that cause us to feel tired. When our bodies need attention, they have few ways to signal that something is wrong short of a total shutdown of a system. Sometimes fatigue is a cry for help.

Says Dr. Rob Krakovitz in his book *High Energy:*

> All mental, emotional, and spiritual problems are eventually manifested or expressed physically. Our physical ills are sometimes an expression of some bottled-up emotion or strong feeling that we can't seem to let out in any other way. The commonly used phrase "sick and tired" comes to mind. People who habitually use this expression are truly sick and tired—the thing they claim to be sick and tired of is only secondary. Don't become emotionally dependent or attached to your fatigue.[2]

Pulling the covers over our heads does not get at the source of the problem. It only masks the root causes of our fatigue. What, besides too little sleep, can cause symptoms of "sleepiness"?

Stress

Stress is perhaps the most overused word of the late twentieth century, but many of us have recognized its potentially disastrous side effects on our health. Stress attacks us on the job, in our relationships, and as we try to balance our growing number of

How Stressful Is Your Life?

Death of spouse	100	____
Divorce	73	____
Marital separation	65	____
Jail term	63	____
Death of a close family member	63	____
Personal injury or illness	53	____
Marriage	50	____
Fired at work	47	____
Marital reconciliation	45	____
Retirement	45	____
Change in health of family member	44	____
Pregnancy	40	____
Sex difficulties	39	____
Gain of new family member	39	____
Business adjustment	39	____
Change in financial state	38	____
Death of a close friend	37	____
Change to a different line of work	36	____
Change in number of arguments with spouse	35	____
Mortgage over one year's net salary	31	____
Foreclosure of mortgage or loan	30	____
Change in responsibilities at work	29	____
Son or daughter leaving home	29	____
Trouble with in-laws	29	____

roles. It makes us feel tense, it helps us overeat, it interferes with our abilities to relate openly to other people, and some doctors say that it lowers our resistance to everything from the common cold to cancer.

When we feel especially "stressed out" we seek escape routes, and sleep is often one of them. But times of stress typically are times of poor sleep. Seneca observed, "Night brings our troubles to light rather than banishes them." We lie awake worrying and sometimes even awaken during the night feeling anxious. The next day we may blame our fatigue on lack of sleep; but a great contributing factor is the stress that caused our poor sleep and is also sapping us of physical and mental strength.

When Dr. Ernest Hartmann studied 500 "variable" sleepers, he

Outstanding personal achievement	28	____
Spouse begins or stops work	26	____
Begin or end school	26	____
Change in living conditions	25	____
Revision of personal habits	24	____
Trouble with boss	23	____
Change in work hours or conditions	20	____
Change in residence	20	____
Change in schools	20	____
Change in recreation	19	____
Change in church activities	19	____
Change in social activities	18	____
Mortgage or loan less than one year's net salary	17	____
Change in sleeping habits	16	____
Change in number of family get-togethers	15	____
Change in eating habits	15	____
Vacation	13	____
Christmas	12	____
Minor violations of the law	11	____
ENTER YOUR TOTAL HERE		____

If your total is over 300, then you have an 80 percent probability of a serious change in your health within the next year.

found that "they needed less sleep when their lives were without change or stress, when they were happy and healthy and involved in interesting or enjoyable tasks."[3]

Illness

There are two types of illness that may cause us to feel tired. The first is the run-of-the-mill cold or flu, which can knock us off our feet totally for a day or two and leave us dragging for a week or more. Our bodies use increased amounts of energy when we have a fever, or when our immune systems are activated to fight a virus. During these times we *do* need more hours of rest, and sleeping more helps the body conserve energy and use it to fight disease.

The Epstein-Barr Virus

The Epstein-Barr virus is often found in people who have severe, persistent fatigue associated with one or more of the following:

- Recurrent low-grade fevers
- Persistent sore throats
- Feelings of depression
- Recurrent headaches
- Muscle and bone pain
- Sleep disturbances
- Lymph node swelling

But feeling fatigued for more than a week or two after other symptoms have passed is cause for concern and a trip to the doctor. Such illnesses as "walking pneumonia" may have found a cordial host in your body, and feeling tired is one way for you to know that treatment is needed.

The other type of illness that can cause fatigue is more serious. Certain forms of cancer, such as leukemia, are sometimes discovered because they cause such overwhelming fatigue.

The Epstein-Barr virus, which may be responsible for mononucleosis, may also be responsible for a wide range of illnesses, some of which are virtually debilitating. The virus tends to attack young adults who are normally energetic, but soon can't even get out of bed in the morning.[4] People who suffer from these types of illness are still exhausted after as much as 20 hours of sleep. Obviously, few doctors consider lack of sleep to be the culprit in this type of fatigue.

Seasonal Affectiveness Disorder (SAD)

Although Seasonal Affectivenes Disorder (SAD) is not a disease per se, it is a problem that affects a very high percentage of people during the winter months. It is most common in northern climates and during the months of November through February, and it is sometimes called "the hibernation response." Symptoms include chronic fatigue, depression, weight gain, irritability, loss of interest in work and sex, and a craving for carbohydrates.[5]

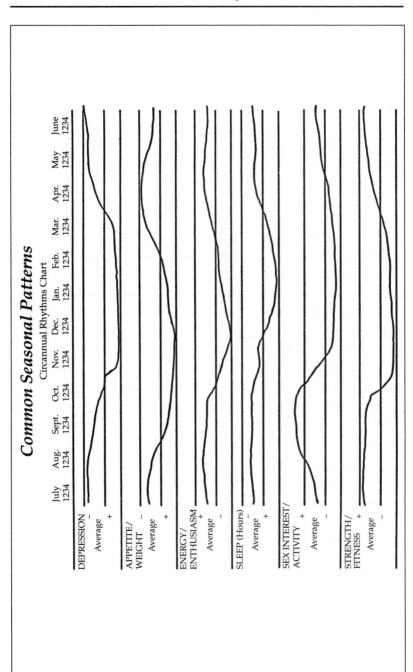

Common Seasonal Patterns

Circannual Rhythms Chart

SAD seems to be caused by our instinctive response to dropping temperatures and lack of light. In an effort to conserve the body's energy, we "hibernate," at least to the degree that modern men and women can. One of the ways we get our natural cues for when to sleep and when to awaken is through our circadian clock. As we discussed in the last chapter, our circadian clock is something like the thermostat in our homes. As our body temperature begins to drop in the evenings, we get the natural cue that it is time to go to bed. As our temperature rises in the morning, we will awaken, even without an alarm. Our circadian clock is reset by changes in light. And that is a major problem for those of us who live in places where the winter months mean fewer hours of light than during the rest of the year.

The cures for SAD include light therapy, exercise, and diet changes. They also include getting less sleep and using the additional time for exposure to artificial light. Ironically, *sleeping more in the winter only aggravates the situation.* If you think you might suffer from SAD, you might consider ordering a light box from one of the companies listed in the Appendix. These special lights are portable and provide very intense light. They are reported to help overcome the symptoms of SAD when used for as little as an hour each day.

Poor Nutrition

How ironic that most of us can buy whatever foods we want, yet we are to a great degree malnourished. We eat fatty foods that are energy sappers and have only passing interest in complex carbohydrates, fruits, and vegetables, which would help us feel more energetic and enable us to control our weight. How many overweight people do you know who seem to be bursting with energy? The fact is that overeating and eating the wrong types of foods make us feel sluggish and what many would call "sleepy." But sleep has nothing to do with our weariness.

In *Women and Fatigue* Dr. Holly Atkinson states that poor nutrition is one of the greatest contributors to fatigue. "Although

American women rarely connect fatigue with eating, either the lack of food or too much of the wrong kind can be an important cause of fatigue."[6]

And it's not true of just women. My husband typically runs out the door in the morning, gulping a cup of coffee. His lunch is either a quick bite on the run or a heavy meal and dessert during a meeting in a restaurant. He eats dinner late—often after 7 P.M.—and follows it with an evening snack. This is not the eating pattern of a person who wants to feel energetic.

Nutrition rarely gets taught in medical school, according to the Committee on Nutrition in Medical Education of the National Research Council. In a survey of U.S. medical schools, it found that fewer than one-quarter of all U.S. medical schools required even one course in nutrition. So such problems as food allergies, which can lead to poor sleep patterns, are rarely discovered in a routine physical exam. If you feel droopy during the average day, take a look at your diet. Seek the help of a qualified nutritionist. You may find that you are allergic to a staple in your diet and fatigue is one of the symptoms.

Other obvious culprits in our diets are alcohol and caffeine. Most of us know better than to drink coffee right before going to bed if we have trouble sleeping, but what is not so obvious is that the mid-afternoon cup of coffee may remain in your system as long as 7 hours. That could either cause problems in going to sleep or cause sleep disturbances, such as inhibiting deep sleep.

"Alcoholism often disturbs the sleep mechanism permanently . . ."

Alcohol may help you feel sleepy, but drink too much and the sleep you get will be of poor quality. Although a glass of wine with dinner probably won't affect most people's sleep, those who drink a great deal or who suffer from alcoholism have chronically impaired sleep. "The typical alcoholic awakens many times during the night, changes rapidly from one stage of sleep to the next. . . . Tragically, alcoholism often disturbs the sleep mechanism permanently, even long after successful withdrawal has occurred," says Richard Trubo in *How to Get a Good Night's Sleep*.[7]

Another reason for feeling tired may be because the foods you eat contain a great amount of the natural amino acid L-tryptophan.* The conventional wisdom that a warm glass of milk will help you sleep is nutritionally backed up by the fact that milk contains this natural sleep inducer. That's fine if you *want* to sleep. But you may be surprised to discover that your after-lunch slump is worsened by the tuna fish you ate—another food naturally high in tryptophan.

Lack of Exercise

Human beings were not created to be sedentary creatures. We have marvelous muscle systems that atrophy without use. We have the ability to develop strength and stamina, which is wasted if we never push ourselves. We have mechanisms that help us withstand shifts in temperature that would send other creatures into shock and bring on certain death. But if we never break out in a sweat, our body can't use this ingenious system to purify ourselves. Most of us are like seldom-driven Ferraris rusting away in a driveway. We have the potential to be a lean, mean machine. But we aren't coming close to living up to our Maker's ideal for us.

We have learned that exercise is "addictive." This is due in part to the fact that our bodies produce endorphins when we exercise, which give us a natural sense of well-being. But lethargy is addictive, too. When we have a very low level of activity we produce a substance called serotonin. Its message to the brain:

---

*L-Tryptophan tablets, once available in health food stores, were recently removed from the shelves because of concern that they are linked to a potentially fatal blood disorder. Scientists believe the problem is with the processing of the substance into tablet form, not the tryptophan itself, which is a naturally occuring amino acid. There is no reason to avoid foods containing tryptophan except that they may cause drowsiness. But do not take tryptophan in tablet form.

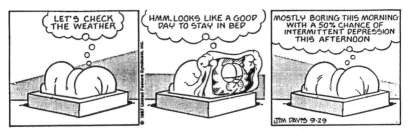

One of the most common reasons for fatigue is depression.

Slow down, feel drowsy, relax. You may feel sleepy and may even doze off. But sleep is just the opposite of what you need. A run around the block would energize you far more than a 15-minute nap.

Depression

A person who has just been fired, gone through a divorce, lost a loved one, or experienced any type of failure, loss, or rejection will often complain of feeling chronically tired. That person is typically suffering from depression, a psychological condition that has physical manifestations such as fatigue. As we all know from personal experience, depression does not occur only after a devastating blow. Sometimes we are less equipped to handle such garden-variety problems as a stalling career, unexciting marriage, or aging body. A psychiatrist might easily identify our problem if we had just lost our job. But his or her task would be more difficult if we simply had been in the same boring job for 10 years and possibly hadn't even admitted to ourselves that the vice presidency was out of reach.

Physical weariness is often a cue to us that something is wrong in our lives—perhaps something that is only known on a subconscious level. Sleep only keeps us from getting to the root of the problem, by "escaping" the evidence.

Pregnancy

Pregnancy is not an illness, but our body sends out signals that are surprisingly similar to the cues it gives us if it is fighting a disease. Instead of fighting off a virus, our body's energy is devoted to growing another human being. The energy required is phenomenal.

When my doctor confirmed that I was pregnant with my first child I was greatly relieved, since I was certain that I was dying of leukemia. No one had prepared me for the exhaustion I felt during my earliest months, and I couldn't imagine that something as natural as pregnancy could have such an effect on my energy level.

During the first trimester of pregnancy a woman will feel "draggy," primarily because of the massive changes taking place in her body. Some doctors believe that a possible explanation for this is that the elevated levels of progesterone present in a woman who is pregnant have a sedative effect.[8] Most women feel better during the next three months, only to grow tired again as the additional weight slows them down. Many women also have difficulty sleeping through the night in the last months, when their size and shape make it difficult to find a comfortable sleeping position.

Rest is important during all stages of pregnancy, and a woman should carefully follow the advice of her obstetrician. But if a woman can't sleep, she should just try to relax and stay off her feet. Lack of sleep will not cause harm to her or her baby, although *a woman who is pregnant or nursing should not consider undertaking an optional program of sleep reduction such as the one outlined in this book.*

Women may also be subject to changes in sleep patterns before menstruation and during menopause. In the first case, hormone changes are suspected to be the cause; in the second, a combination of hormonal changes bringing on hot flashes conspires to awaken a woman during her normal sleeping hours.

Sleep Disorders

As stated earlier, besides lack of sleep, sleep disorders may mean that a person gets as much or more than enough total sleep time, but the sleep itself is disturbed by such problems as sleep apnea. Another problem of the chronically sleepy person who gets an adequate amount of sleep is narcolepsy. Although this is sometimes depicted comically on television, the tendency to fall asleep at inappropriate times is a very serious physical disorder and is not necessarily related to the amount of sleep a person gets at night. Anyone who suffers from snoring or gasping while asleep, has uncontrolled movements, such as regular kicking, or falls asleep at inappropriate times should see a physician. These could be symptoms of serious, even life-threatening, disorders.

Prescription Drugs

Many drugs that are prescribed for a variety of ailments also cause sleep disturbances. Some prescription and over-the-counter drugs actually contain caffeine. Others, such as antihistamines, tranquilizers, muscle relaxants, and even diuretics, cause drowsiness. If you regularly take any type of medication, be sure to read the literature that accompanies it to determine whether drowsiness or excitability are possible side effects.

Take Control

Assuming that you are not ill or pregnant, you can take steps to overcome the tiredness you may feel. And if you don't typically feel tired, you're ahead of the game. You will have an easier time cutting back your sleep and maintaining a life-style that includes more hours for living, not escaping.

**You can control your sleep;
your sleep does not control you.**

The most important thing to remember is that *your sleep does not have to control you.* Still skeptical? You may appreciate a study done by sleep researchers who observed three groups of people of relatively similar backgrounds. They removed all evidence of time from them, including clocks, light, and temperature change. Then they had each group sleep exactly 8 hours. The only difference was in the information they gave each group. The first was told they were being sleep deprived, and were only allowed to sleep 6 hours. The second group was told that they had slept 10 hours. The third group was told the truth. The first group complained of sleepiness, irritability, and impaired concentration. The second group complained of lethargy. The third group reported that they felt fine.

The need for sleep is not *all* in our heads. But for many of us, sleep, to a certain degree, is a learned dependency or a comfortable habit. There is nothing wrong with the amount of sleep we get unless we want to do more with our lives. Just half an hour each day would add more than 182 hours of living in a year. That's the equivalent of an extra month of work weeks. Isn't it worth finding out if this incredible resource is available to you?

SLEEPFACT: Dolphins demonstrate very sophisticated sleep patterns. First the right half of their brain sleeps; then the left. They are never totally unconscious.

Chapter Four

Step 1: Self-Assessment

Dost thou love life? Then do not squander time; for that's
the stuff life is made of.

—Benjamin Franklin

I had nearly missed the airplane, and as I hurriedly stowed my briefcase beneath the seat in front of me and fastened my seat belt as the plane began to roll away from the gate. I couldn't help thinking that this incident was a perfect metaphor for my life: It seemed to be taking off with me barely aboard.

The demands of my business were growing to the point that I didn't think a 12-hour work day would be enough to accomplish all I had to do. My children needed more attention and the extracurricular activities of my older son meant that weekends and early evenings were regularly booked. My husband had just taken over a major area in his firm and not only did he work long hours, but he was under terrific stress. Our time together was confined to the few hours after the children went to bed, while we either did additional work or collapsed and watched a mindless television show. Our lives were full, but the quality of life was low for all of us.

Something had to give, I knew, but I just didn't see a way out except through major surgery on some area of my life. I thought about my friend who had 2 more hours in his day. I knew what I had learned through my sleep research. But I also knew how I felt. Could I really reduce my sleep during a time when I was so out of control?

I felt tired all the time anyway, even though I was getting 8 hours of sleep each night. Maybe I wouldn't feel that much worse with a little less sleep, I reasoned. And perhaps the extra time would help me get my life in balance. So with a sense of *What do I have to lose?* I decided to apply what I had learned to my own life.

But how was I going to go about it? I pulled out a piece of paper and did what I had learned to do in my business training. I wrote my goal across the top of the page:

GOAL: To bring balance to my life

Just seeing the words on paper gave me some hope. Balance was what I was seeking. But soon the doubts flooded in. *How could I ever break the hectic cycle I was in?* I forced myself to think through what I had learned about sleep. Then I wrote down my possible solution: *Sleep less; use "extra" time to relieve stress.*

Once again, based on my business training, I knew it was important to find out exactly where things stood. I began to feel overwhelmed until I methodically wrote it all down on paper. The questions I asked myself became the components of the first step in my personal sleep management plan.

Five Questions to Help You Assess Your Sleep Needs

If you've come this far, you may be tempted to skip this step and move right on to implementing the program. But self-assessment is an important step for both medical and motivational reasons. Most of us think we know a great deal about our own sleep. But I found that I had nearly as many misconceptions about my own sleep as I had about sleep in general. And I knew that I might be able to find ways not only to reduce the amount of sleep I needed, but also to improve the sleep I was getting.

1. What Are Your Current Sleep Patterns?

Because so many people complain about sleep problems, it is important to have a "sleep checkup" before you go any further. Answer the questions below to help you gain an understanding of your current sleep patterns:

During weekdays, I sleep approximately____ hours per night.

On weekends, I sleep approximately____ hours per night.

For the most part, I feel
- ❑ well rested during the day
- ❑ occasionally tired during the day
- ❑ often tired during the day
- ❑ exhausted during the day

On weekend days I feel
- ❑ better
- ❑ worse
- ❑ about the same

On the average, I fall asleep
- ❑ in less than 10 minutes
- ❑ in 10 to 30 minutes
- ❑ in 30 minutes to 1 hour
- ❑ in 1 hour or longer from the time I go to bed

Once I am asleep, I awaken
- ❑ only when I hear a loud noise or when physically roused
- ❑ when I hear occasional noises or minor disturbances
- ❑ once in a while, for no apparent reason
- ❑ about once a night, for no apparent reason
- ❑ more than once a night

If I awaken at night, I fall back to sleep
- ❑ almost immediately
- ❑ in 10 minutes or less
- ❑ after 10 minutes to 30 minutes
- ❑ after a long time
- ❑ rarely at all

When I awaken in the morning, I
- ❑ jump out of bed and am ready to go
- ❑ get up fairly quickly
- ❑ lie in bed for up to 15 minutes
- ❑ lie in bed for as long as I can—more than 15 minutes
- ❑ fall back to sleep and sleep as long as I can

I am told that I snore
- ❑ not at all
- ❑ when I have a cold
- ❑ occasionally
- ❑ regularly

When my parents were my age, they slept

Father	Mother	
❑	❑	more than 8 hours each night
❑	❑	approximately 7 to 8 hours each night
❑	❑	approximately 6 to 7 hours each night
❑	❑	approximately 5 to 6 hours each night
❑	❑	less than 5 hours nightly

I know that one or both of my parents suffer(ed) from sleep disorders including
- ❑ insomnia
- ❑ malsomnia
- ❑ narcolepsy
- ❑ hypersomnia
- ❑ sleep apnea
- ❑ sleepwalking
- ❑ sleep talking
- ❑ other_____

What can you learn about yourself from doing this sleep history? First, you can understand more about your sleep. For example, I discovered that I averaged 8 hours sleep per night on weekdays, but 9 or more hours on weekend nights. When I thought about it, I discovered that I usually felt groggy on weekends. This was my first clue that I could be getting too much sleep, not too little. I was also pleased to discover that I was a relatively sound sleeper with few sleep disturbances.

Does it take you more than 10 minutes to fall asleep? Do you lie awake worrying about problems at the office or at home? If so, you are dealing with stressful situations that may be draining your energy. You may have developed a nighttime worry habit where you automatically get into bed, review the day's events, and then begin to fret. This type of routine not only robs you of sleep, it causes you to be tense and may lead to poor sleep throughout the night.

Try to find a way to deal with your problems before they rob you of your health. Some people find that daily vigorous exercise gives them an outlet and helps relieve tension. Perhaps you will want to see a professional counselor who can help you deal with your problems.

In his classic book, *How to Stop Worrying and Start Living*, Dale Carnegie recommends that you ask yourself, "What's the worst that could happen?" He then recommends that you prepare yourself for it. I find that this question helps me deal directly with hidden concerns. Since I took the advice in this book I rarely have a hard time falling asleep.

Barbara Walters's nighttime routine includes making a to-do list for the next day. Having committed everything to writing, she claims to fall asleep easily knowing that she will be able to start right in on the work she needs to do the next morning.

If you routinely stay awake for half an hour or more every night, you may think of yourself as an insomniac. You may simply be a naturally shorter sleeper. A simple way to deal with your "problem" is to assess how long it typically takes you to fall asleep, then cut your time in bed back by that amount. For example, if you are still awake 45 minutes after going to bed, do not get into bed for 45 minutes after your normal bedtime. After a few days of doing this, you should be falling asleep soon after you get into bed. If you want, you can then get into bed at a slightly earlier time. But if you don't fall asleep fairly quickly, get up and read or do something relaxing.

In fact, one of the simplest and most widely prescribed methods of treating insomnia is sleep restriction. Doctors theorize that people who sleep poorly are often sleeping inefficiently. After several nights of cutting back on your sleep, your body will begin to learn to make the most of its time in bed. Not only will you begin to fall asleep more quickly, you will sleep more deeply.

Doctors theorize that people who sleep poorly are often sleeping inefficiently.

Do you typically sleep through the night? Or are you awakened spontaneously? If you wake up once or twice a night you should first assess your environment. Is something disturbing you, such as noise, light, the movement of your spouse? If there are no outside factors, analyze your own routine and diet. Do you take sleeping pills? They may help you fall asleep, but they do not help you sleep deeply and may contribute to nighttime awakenings. Do you drink alcohol at night? You may feel relaxed and sleepy after a glass of wine, but alcohol disturbs sleep more than it acts as a sleep inducer. Coffee, colas, chocolate, and other caffeinated foods and beverages may not bother you when it comes to falling asleep, but they can affect how well you sleep. Chapter 9 examines factors that contribute to efficient sleep. You may want to review these factors to help improve your sleep.

Do you jump out of bed in the morning, fully awake and ready to go? If so, you are in the minority. You will probably find the sleep management plan relatively easy to follow and may not need as much sleep as you think you do.

If you are a chronic snorer, you should see your doctor, who may refer you to an eye, ear, nose, and throat specialist. You may have a sinus problem; you may also suffer from a sleep-related breathing disorder, such as sleep apnea.

What do the sleep patterns of your parents have to do with you? Plenty, it seems. Sleep patterns and disorders may be hereditary, just as other tendencies are inherited. First, we probably learn our attitudes about sleep from our parents, which then affects our views. But we may also be naturally short sleepers if our parents are. Or we may inherit their ability to take catnaps.

2. What Are Your Personal Rhythms?

"Are you an owl or a lark?" When I mentioned that I was writing about sleep, this was one of the most common questions people asked me. Almost everyone had an opinion as to where they stood on the subject, although research indicates that only about 10 percent of the population is extremely predisposed in one direction or the other. If you are curious about your own tendencies, take the survey on the following pages.

If you find that your score indicates you are a moderate morning or evening type, you are like most people. If you are neither type, you can probably shift your sleeping patterns either way. But if you are definitely a morning or evening type, you may be the type of person who has a very hard time adjusting when flying into different time zones or when changing to a different shift.

We all have distinct natural rhythms that give us optimum times of day for productivity as well as "down times." These times are linked to our circadian clocks. We also learn to adapt more or less to what is expected of us in our environment. My friend the writer, whom I mentioned in chapter 1, finds that his most productive, creative time occurs after 10 P.M. I wouldn't trust my ability to write a complete sentence at that time, but I find that the ideas flow for me before 10 A.M.

If you are really serious about finding your optimum times, you might consider tracking your body temperature using a basal thermometer. If you take your temperature every waking hour for a day or two, you will probably find that you have a pattern of rising temperature in the morning, then falling temperature until

Owl and Lark Questionnaire

Instructions:
1. Please read each question very carefully before answering.
2. Answer ALL questions.
3. Answer questions in numerical order.
4. Each question should be answered independently of others. Do NOT go back and check your answers.
5. All questions have a selection of answers. For each question place a cross alongside ONE answer only. Some questions have a scale instead of a selection of answers. Place a cross at the appropriate point along the scale.

1. Considering only your own "feeling best" rhythm, at what time would you get up if you were entirely free to plan your day?

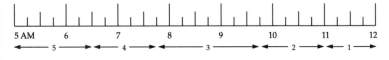

2. Considering only your own "feeling best" rhythm, at what time would you go to bed if you were entirely free to plan your evening?

3. If there is a specific time at which you have to get up in the morning, to what extent are you dependent on being woken up by an alarm clock?
   ❑ 4 Not at all dependent   ❑ 3 Slightly dependent
   ❑ 2 Fairly dependent   ❑ 1 Very dependent

4. Assuming adequate environmental conditions, how easy do you find getting up in the mornings?
   ❑ 1 Not at all easy   ❑ 2 Not very easy
   ❑ 3 Fairly easy   ❑ 4 Very easy

5. How alert do you feel during the first half hour after having woken in the mornings?
   ❑ 1 Not at all alert   ❑ 2 Slightly alert
   ❑ 3 Fairly alert   ❑ 4 Very alert

6. How is your appetite during the first half hour after having woken in the morning?

   ❏ 1 Very poor   ❏ 2 Fairly poor

   ❏ 3 Fairly good   ❏ 4 Very good

7. During the first half-hour after having woken in the morning, how tired do you feel?

   ❏ 1 Very tired   ❏ 2 Fairly tired

   ❏ 3 Fairly refreshed   ❏ 4 Very refreshed

8. When you have no commitments the next day, at what time do you go to bed compared to your usual bedtime?

   ❏ 4 Seldom or never later   ❏ 3 Less than one hour later

   ❏ 2 1–2 hours later   ❏ 1 More than two hours later

9. You have decided to engage in some physical exercise. A friend suggests that you do this one hour twice a week and the best time for him is between 7:00 and 8:00 A.M. Bearing in mind nothing else but your own "feeling best" rhythm, how do you think you would perform?

   ❏ 4 Would be in good form   ❏ 3 Would be in reasonable form

   ❏ 2 Would find it difficult ❏ 1 Would find it very difficult

10. At what time in the evening do you feel tired and as a result in need of sleep?

| 8 PM | 9 | 10 | 11 | 12 AM | 1 | 2 | 3 |

←— 5 —→ ←— 4 —→ ←——— 3 ———→ ←— 2 —→ ←— 1 —→

11. You wish to be at your peak performance for a test which you know is going to be mentally exhausting and lasting for two hours. You are entirely free to plan your day and considering only your own "feeling best" rhythm, which ONE of the four testing times would you choose?

    ❏ 6 8:00–10:00 A.M.   ❏ 4 11:00 A.M.–1:00 P.M.

    ❏ 2 3:00–5:00 P.M.   ❏ 0 7:00–9:00 P.M.

12. If you went to bed at 11:00 P.M. at what level of tiredness would you be?

    ❏ 0 Not at all tired   ❏ 2 A little tired

    ❏ 5 Fairly tired   ❏ 9 Very tired

13. For some reason you have gone to bed several hours later than usual, but there is no need to get up at any particular time the next morning. Which ONE of the following events are you most likely to experience?

❑ 4 Will wake up at usual time and will NOT fall asleep

❑ 3 Will wake up at usual time and will doze thereafter

❑ 2 Will wake up at usual time but will fall asleep again

❑ 1 Will NOT wake up until later than usual

14. One night you have to remain awake between 4:00–6:00 A.M. in order to carry out a night watch. You have no commitments the next day. Which ONE of the following alternatives will suit you best?

❑ 2 Would NOT go to bed until watch was over

❑ 1 Would take a nap before and sleep after

❑ 3 Would take a good sleep before and nap after

❑ 4 Would take ALL sleep before watch

15. You have to do two hours of hard physical work. You are entirely free to plan your day. Considering only your own "feeling best" rhythm, which ONE of the following times would you choose?

❑ 4 8:00–10:00 A.M.

❑ 3 11:00 A.M.–1:00 P.M.

❑ 2 3:00–5:00 P.M.

❑ 1 7:00–9:00 P.M.

16. You have decided to engage in hard physical exercise. A friend suggests that you do this for one hour twice a week and the best time for him is between 10:00–11:00 P.M. Bearing in mind nothing else but your own "feeling best" rhythm, how well do you think you would perform?

❑ 1 Would be in good form

❑ 2 Would be in reasonable form

❑ 3 Would find it difficult

❑ 4 Would find it very difficult

17. Suppose that you can choose your own work hours. Assume that you worked a FIVE-hour day (including breaks) and that your job was interesting and paid by results. Which FIVE CONSECUTIVE HOURS would you select?

12 1 2 3 4 5 6 7 8 9 10 11 12 1 2 3 4 5 6 7 8 9 10 11 12
MIDNIGHT   NOON   MIDNIGHT

◄— 1 —►◄— 5 —►◄ 4 ◄— 3 —►◄ 2 ►◄———— 1 ————►

18. At what time of the day do you think that you reach your "feeling best" peak?

12 1 2 3 4 5 6 7 8 9 10 11 12 1 2 3 4 5 6 7 8 9 10 11 12
MIDNIGHT   NOON   MIDNIGHT

◄—— 1 ——► ◄— 5 —►◄— 4 —►◄——— 3 ———►◄——— 2 ———►◄— 1 —►

19. One hears about "morning" and "evening" types of people. Which ONE of these types do you consider yourself to be?

❏ 6 Definitely a "morning" type

❏ 4 Rather more a "morning" than an "evening" type

❏ 2 Rather more an "evening" than a "morning type"

❏ 0 Definitely an "evening" type

Scoring For questions 3, 4, 5, 6, 7, 8, 9, 11, 12, 13, 14, 15, 16, and 19, the appropriate score for each response is displayed beside the answer box.

For questions 1, 2, 10, and 18, the cross made along each scale is referred to the appropriate score value range below the scale. For question 17 the most extreme cross on the right hand side is taken as the reference point and the appropriate score value range below this point is taken.

The scores are added together and the sum converted into a five-point Morningness-Eveningness scale:

	Score
Definitely Morning Type	70–86
Moderately Morning Type	59–69
Neither Type	42–58
Moderately Evening Type	31–41
Definitely Evening Type	16–30

mid-afternoon. Your temperature will probably rise again into early evening, then fall off, signaling bedtime. This exercise may be helpful to you in scheduling your time for optimum productivity. But what if you are not able to adapt your schedule to your natural time?

In *Wide Awake at 3:00 A.M.* Richard Coleman points out that we may have made a mistake in not respecting our natural rhythms. Shift workers, especially those who work between 3 A.M. and 6 A.M., have the most difficulty staying awake and have the most accidents on the job. If you have any doubts about the severity of the problems that can occur consider that the Chernobyl, Three-Mile Island, and Bhopal disasters all occurred in the early morning hours and were attributed to human error.

Or consider this chilling error:

A few years ago a Boeing 707 was scheduled to fly into Los Angeles International Airport shortly after midnight. The flight and crew had originated in New York, so that for the crew it was now about 3 A.M., the low point on the circadian alertness cycle. As the plane approached LAX, the air traffic controllers were amazed to see it maintaining its 32,000-foot altitude. Repeated descent clearances were ignored by the three-man flight crew. The situation became more perplexing and dangerous as the 707 overshot the airport and flew 50 miles out over the Pacific Ocean on a dwindling fuel supply. Not until it was 100 miles out over the Pacific were the controllers finally able to awaken the three sleeping pilots—who were cruising on automatic pilot—by triggering a series of chimes in the cockpit. At that point the aircraft had just enough fuel to return safely to Los Angeles.[1]

You may find that you have monthly as well as daily rhythms. Men and women both experience hormonal changes that may affect sleep patterns. Some women find that sleepiness is one aspect of Premenstrual Syndrome. This is not just an emotional response to hormonal changes. A sleep laboratory study found that women who complained of excessive sleepiness before menstruation were in many cases getting very little Stage 3 or 4 sleep.[2] No one knows why this is true, but without this deep sleep a person will feel tired. If you observe this in your own life, you may want to anticipate it and plan around it, although there is really very little that can be done. Sleeping longer will probably do little to improve your chances of getting the deep sleep you need.

3. What Are Your Attitudes about Life?

The question, "How do you feel about life?" may seem odd, but your view of life in general carries over very directly to your beliefs about sleep. Many books have been published recently about the ability of the mind to control the body. These books, such as Dr. Bernie Siegel's *Love, Medicine and Miracles*, show how the power of positive thinking can sometimes successfully heal the body of diseases such as cancer.

"We don't yet understand all the ways in which brain chemicals are related to emotions and thoughts, but the salient point is that our state of mind has an immediate and direct effect on our state of body. We can change the body by dealing with how we feel."[3]

If the mind can actually combat disease,
it must also be able to play a key role
in reshaping sleep patterns.

If the mind can actually combat disease, it must also be able to play a key role in reshaping sleep patterns. According to the AMA's book *Guide to Better Sleep,* some of us need less sleep when things are going well and more sleep when life is tough. A study cited in the same book compared long sleepers and short sleepers and found that "The short-sleepers tended to be efficient, energetic, and ambitious. . . . The long-sleepers, as a group, showed more doubts about their career choices and life situations. . . ."[4]

If severely depriving a person of sleep can break a cycle of depression, and if short sleepers appear to be more energetic and "up" than long sleepers, doesn't it seem that our attitudes can be affected by our sleep and vice versa?.

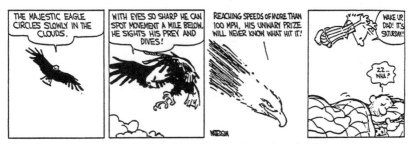

Our sleep patterns are often affected by other members of our family.

A year ago I would have said that less sleep would distinctly worsen my attitude about life. Without 8 hours I would feel irritable, grumpy, and pessimistic. But a year after implementing my sleep management plan I find that I am much more positive about life and significantly more energetic. I'm sure that one of the main reasons for this is that I spend much of my new-found time in stress-reducing activities. But the people I have interviewed who sleep less than 7 hours a night do seem to share a certain optimism and energy that is missing from the over-8-hours-a-night sleepers.

Without a careful study it is impossible to determine which came first, the short nights or the optimistic attitude. But I know that, in my own case at least, cutting back sleep improved my outlook.

4. How Regular Is Your Schedule?

Some of us live our lives very predictably. In bed by 11 P.M., up at 7 A.M., we rarely deviate from the schedule. Others work late or are up with the baby or travel across time zones. Just how much you can control your time is something only you can determine. Begin to be aware of the exact time you go to bed and awaken. What factors affect these times? For example, do you stay up to watch the news or predictions for the next day's weather?

Do you travel across time zones more than once a month? If so, you may find that you suffer the effects of jet lag much of the time. You probably find that adjusting to westbound travel is easier than adjusting to eastbound travel. You may also find that jet lag may be lessened to some degree by diet.

Jet lag was more of a problem for me before I began to manage my sleep. Perhaps this is because I had more adjusting to do with 8 hours of sleep than with 6½ hours of sleep. For whatever reason, I was pleasantly surprised to discover that the side effects of jet lag were minimal after I had been on the sleep management plan for a month, and were almost nonexistent after a few months of consistently managing my sleep.

Whether you travel or not, the regularity of your hours will have an effect on how tired you feel. As we learned, the body's "sleepostat" is a device that takes its cue from the previous day's information. If you stay up until 1 A.M. on Friday and Saturday nights, then sleep in until 9 A.M. or 10 A.M. the next morning, don't be surprised if you are wide awake at midnight on Sunday night and more exhausted than usual when your alarm goes off at 7 A.M. Monday morning. You have begun to reprogram your body to be on a different time zone over the weekend. Suddenly you expect it to snap back to a different routine on Monday.

5. What Are the Attitudes of Others?

If you are married, your sleep patterns are heavily influenced by your spouse. But you are also influenced by children, roommates, and neighbors. I have two boys, one a lark and the other an owl. The lark cheerfully awakens with the sun and sings and plays until I come to get him in the morning. By 7:30 P.M. he begins to ask to go to bed and almost always falls asleep immediately. My other son, however, would gladly stay up until midnight and often lies awake for an hour or more at night. In order to get him up and to school on time I literally drag him out of bed in the morning. Clearly, I can't just choose my own ideal schedule. And since my husband loves to sleep in, I often take the boys downstairs on weekends to let him have some extra sleep.

We are not only influenced by the people we live with, but also by the attitudes of people around us. I was surprised to find how many people are "closet" short sleepers. They don't talk about their sleep patterns because they feel abnormal.

In a wonderful column entitled "In Praise of Cheerful Early Risers," Ellen Goodman tells of her own experience:

> Most people do not consider dawn to be an attractive experience—unless they are still up. Most people are congenitally unable to smile before 9:00 A.M. . . . By my mid-twenties I learned that I would never be popular if I continued to wake people up early with fresh insights, or if I continued to sing while I squeezed orange juice. . . . So, sad to say, I became closety. I learned to pass. I learned to lie still until 8:30 A.M. If I was caught with open eyes at 6:00 or 7:00, I blamed it on insomnia.[5]

You may find you are influenced by the people in your profession, or even the part of the country in which you live. New Yorkers tend to hate breakfast meetings and often start work at 9:30 A.M. Midwesterners, as a group, are early risers. Restaurants are bustling at 7:30 A.M. and many businesses open at 8 A.M. On the West Coast customs vary by type of business. Those in companies linked to the East Coast (such as stockbrokers) are often at the office very early. Westerners generally tend to observe slightly earlier hours than easterners, but not as early as midwesterners.

Setting your own patterns may seem difficult at first. But if you are feeling bored with life—or overly challenged—changing your schedule can be an exciting way to open new opportunities. You may find that watching the sunrise gives you a new lease on life. Or you may discover that staying up to watch Johnny Carson gives you just the shot of humor you need.

SLEEPFACT: The ancient poet Lausius felt that 5 hours was enough sleep for young and old men; 6 for merchants; 7 for aristocrats; and 8 for "the lazy and wholly idle man."

Chapter Five

Step 2: Motivation

Sleeping is no mean art: for its sake one must stay
awake all day.
—Friedrich Nietzsche

Some people, I am told, hop gleefully out of bed in the morning and never look back. And then there are the rest of us—those who moan and groan and bargain with our alarm clocks for "just 10 more minutes." We snuggle further into our cocoons, trying to savor those last delicious moments before we face the cold, cruel world.

For that first kind of person, motivation may be a small part of the sleep management plan. But the majority of us need both short- and long-term reasons for disengaging ourselves from the comfort of our beds, especially on cold winter days when pulling back the covers is a physically painful experience.

What Motivates You?

During the period of time when I was doing research on sleep, my husband was interested and attentive as I discussed my discoveries. But when I began to experiment on myself in an attempt to reduce my sleeping hours, he was both amused and skeptical. "Why bother?" was his reaction. Tom is the sort of orderly, paced person who seems to accomplish exactly what he needs to do. The idea of having more time was a curiosity rather than a fantasy to him.

For me, just the idea of having extra time in my day gave me a boost. I quickly began to imagine all of the things I could do. I fantasized about projects I could accomplish. I let myself pull out of storage all of those dreams I had put in mothballs because I was too busy dealing with daily life. I savored the thought of time for myself—time that was not stolen from family or work, but time that I could enjoy guilt free.

Tom and I have very different personalities and are motivated in very different ways. I knew that jumping out of bed earlier each day would not be easy, but I could immediately recognize the benefits. Tom, on the other hand, could not imagine anything enticing him out of bed a minute earlier than necessary. By our basic personalities, I was a much better candidate for the sleep management plan than Tom was.

Cutting the total hours you sleep, whether by subtracting time from the evening or morning hours, is not an easy, comfortable thing to do. It takes some discipline, and I will suggest crutches for you to use. It feels a bit uncomfortable at first, but you may be surprised at how quickly that discomfort is replaced by an improved sense of well-being. It may even seem a little unusual to friends who, like my husband, can't see a need for more time. But sleep management is not aimed at cutting out sleep just to see if you can do it. We're talking about trade-offs.

The sleep management plan is not really about sleeping; it's about living.

Only you know how you want to live your life. It's not worth cutting back on your sleep if you don't value the extra time you're given. If you're like my husband, you probably shouldn't undertake this program. Enjoy your time in bed. But if the idea of quiet time alone for reading, writing, exercising, meditating, working on a hobby, or getting a head start on the day is enticing, you have the motivation needed to successfully embark on this program.

When I began to talk to people I knew about the sleep plan their responses were as diverse as the people themselves and often provided new insight into people I thought I knew well.

My friend Jill, for example, got a dreamy look in her eye when I told her that it was possible to add extra time to every day. "I always wanted to be a sculptor," she said. "That would give me time to pursue my dream."

John, my all-business co-worker, immediately saw the benefits: "That would give me time to catch up on my professional journals and pursue some of the projects that could lead to my next promotion!"

Marion, the mother of three small children had more basic desires. "Just think . . . time to myself, alone in the bathtub."

Several friends cited neglected exercise programs they would be able to incorporate into their lives if they had extra time. One woman said she fantasized about going to the grocery store early in the morning before there were any lines at the checkout counter. A man I met on an airplane said that he'd be able to study Italian, a life-long dream.

Your dreams may be as ambitious as starting your own company or as personally meaningful as having time alone to think. Whatever they are, you can come closer to them by having extra time in each day.

In the last chapter you did a sleep checkup to help learn more about where you are today. Now it's time to think more about where you want to be tomorrow. A good place to start is with a "time pie." Use it to determine your current use of time, as well as your desired use of time.

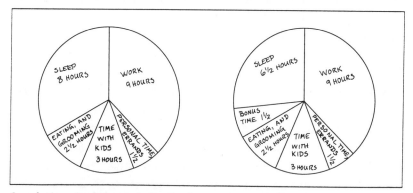

Sample time pies, before and after the sleep management plan.

How to Find More Time in Your Day

1. Reduce the number of hours you watch television.
2. Find a way to commute to work that allows you to read, or listen to tapes while you drive.
3. Use your lunch hour once a week for a specific activity.
4. Trade child-care services with another mother.
5. Simplify your grooming.
6. Cut your wardrobe down to the essentials and decide the night before what you are going to wear the next day.
7. Make a priority list each day and do the important things first.
8. Make a list of 15-minute tasks you can do while waiting for an appointment, or while talking on the telephone.
9. Keep a time log for a week and look for places where you could reclaim 15 minutes here and there throughout your day.
10. Begin the sleep management plan and get an extra 30 minutes to 2 hours each day.

Draw two circles on a sheet of paper. On the first, block out the elements of your day that are predetermined. For example, if you work an 8-hour day and spend 1 hour commuting, 9 hours of weekdays are already accounted for. You will have a certain amount of time committed to meals (probably 1½ to 2½ hours each day). You need to account for grooming time, morning and night. (Women average 1½ hours; men about half that time.) If you are a parent, you will want to account for time with your children. You may also have a daily commitment to exercising, studying, or socializing. Block out the pieces of the pie that are accounted for.

Whatever is left over is *your* time. What would you like to do with it? Take a few minutes to think about the things you currently do with that time. Do you spend hours watching television? Before I did a time pie of my own I would have said that I rarely watched television. But when I analyzed where the hours went I was shocked to find that I spent nearly 2 hours each day in front of the television. I routinely watched a morning news program, then the evening news, a program in the evenings, followed by the local news and weather. I was a television-news junkie and I didn't even know it!

Doing a time pie helped me make better use of the waking hours I already had. That was important motivation to me, because I knew then that there was a real need for more time in my life, and I wanted to use it effectively.

Take a closer look at the time you spend each day on various activities with an eye toward balance. Is your life unbalanced in any direction? Do you have time each day to attend to your own physical, mental, and spiritual growth? Are most of your hours spent at work or attending to the needs of others? How do you actually feel during the various activities of your day—stressed, emotionally exhausted, physically worn out? What needs do you have that are not currently being met?

What to Do with Extra Hours

Perhaps it seems odd to ask what you would do with extra time. We tend to view time like money. We could never have too much of either. But reclaiming extra time in your life is a little like winning the lottery. It might seem like a windfall, but if you don't use the time carefully you can waste the extra time just as easily as you wasted what you had to begin with.

> ***Just an extra 30 minutes a day could change your life if you use it effectively.***

If one of your overriding objectives is to help achieve balance in your life, you have to be careful that the extra time you gain is not simply applied to an already overloaded area, such as work. Achieving a sense of balance in your life will give you more energy, will reduce stress, and will contribute to better health. If you are able to keep this objective in mind as you plan your time, you will be able to enjoy the benefits in every area of your life.

Guidelines
for Using Extra Time

1. DO use the extra time to bring balance to your life.
2. DO something just for you.
3. DON'T feel guilty about how you use this time. You haven't taken it away from anyone else.
4. DO use the time for activities that will help you "de-stress" your life, such as exercise, prayer, meditation.
5. DON'T let anyone else decide where this time should go.
6. DO set a schedule for your extra time.
7. DON'T hesitate to change the schedule if it doesn't suit you.
8. DO adjust to the seasons and change your activities accordingly.
9. DO try to stay on schedule even on weekends.
10. DO dare to explore new dreams.

Based on my experience and the experience of others, I'd suggest you start with short-term goals that have almost immediate payoffs as you plan to use your extra time. Ask yourself, *How could I use the extra time to improve my daily life?*

When you analyzed your life-style, did you find problems that were contributing to fatigue, unrelated to illness? Could you benefit from regular exercise? Would your life seem more balanced if you took some time for prayer, meditation, or journaling? Analyze yourself physically, mentally, emotionally, spiritually. How could you use extra time to specifically heal yourself in any or all these areas?

In Phase I of the sleep plan, you gain an extra 30 minutes daily. That might not seem like much, but it equals 3½ extra hours a week, 14 extra hours a month, or 21 additional 8-hour days a year. Just an extra 30 minutes a day could change your life *if you use it effectively.*

Motivation for staying up later or getting up earlier will be directly tied to how much you believe in the benefits of the extra time you gain. That's why this is such an important step in the program. It is also critical that you treat this time as bonus time. Don't just let your normal activities expand to fill more time. I don't recommend that you use it to do extra work-related activities, either, unless you really enjoy them.

When I analyzed my own life, I found that my lack of exercise was probably a great contributor to my own sense of fatigue. I also knew that without a regular physical activity, I would have a harder time shedding my extra weight.

I also realized that during my day I rarely had time to myself. I was either with my family or my employees, and I felt that my emotional health was impaired at times just by the lack of solitude in my life. In addition, I was feeling "out of control" on many days—a vague emotional sense that I didn't know which end was up, or what was really important in my life. I knew from experience that this signaled a lack of spiritual perspective in my life.

In answer to the question, *What could improve my life tomorrow?* I jotted down on a piece of paper:

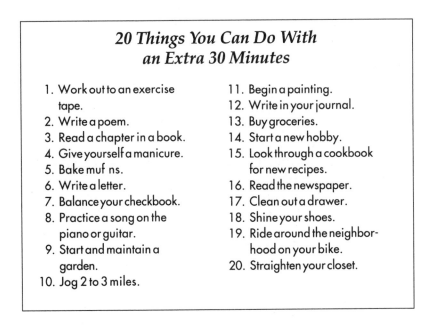

20 Things You Can Do With an Extra 30 Minutes

1. Work out to an exercise tape.
2. Write a poem.
3. Read a chapter in a book.
4. Give yourself a manicure.
5. Bake muf ns.
6. Write a letter.
7. Balance your checkbook.
8. Practice a song on the piano or guitar.
9. Start and maintain a garden.
10. Jog 2 to 3 miles.
11. Begin a painting.
12. Write in your journal.
13. Buy groceries.
14. Start a new hobby.
15. Look through a cookbook for new recipes.
16. Read the newspaper.
17. Clean out a drawer.
18. Shine your shoes.
19. Ride around the neighborhood on your bike.
20. Straighten your closet.

1. Exercise
2. Solitude
3. Spiritual centering
4. Prioritizing my day

You'll want to write your own list of priorities. To get you started, think about how you would complete these statements:

My life would be perfect if _____

_____

If I had 1 extra hour in each day I could _____

_____

If wishing would make it so, I would _____

_____

If I were granted 3 wishes, I would wish for

1. _____

2. _____

3. _____

Go ahead. Imagine a perfect world just for you!

Because the first 30 minutes of sleep reduction are the most important, I would suggest that you write down a specific goal or goals for this phase and then do a schedule for using the time. Specify the exact activity you will undertake, and try to find something you can do every day, rather than alternating days. Remember, you will be altering *either* your bedtime or your wake-up time. It is important to confine your activities to the specific period you are adding to your current schedule.

My specific goals looked like this for the first phase of my sleep plan:

1. I will ride my exercise bicycle for 15 minutes each morning.
2. While riding, I will pray, meditate, and prioritize my day.

3. I will shower and begin to get ready before the rest of the family awakens, giving me time to myself.

My simple schedule looked like this:

6:30 A.M.-6:45 A.M.	Ride bicycle; pray, meditate, prioritize
6:45 A.M.-7:00 A.M.	Shower, do makeup, get ready for day
7:00 A.M.	Awaken rest of family cheerfully

The next chapter details more about how to actually reduce your sleep time. But before you begin to do it, spend a few days *visualizing* what your life will be like with this "bonus" of half an hour a day. *See* yourself feeling more in control of your day. *Feel* the extra energy you will have once you add exercise or meditation to your daily life and rid yourself of some of the destructive stress that is taking its toll.

Set a date, perhaps a few days or a week in the future, when you don't anticipate any major disruptions at work or at home, and when you can reasonably expect to have a fairly consistent schedule for the following few weeks. (Don't try to start the program right before or right after a vacation or a major holiday when routines tend to be disrupted.) Call it "B Day"—for the *bonus* time you will begin to enjoy from that day on.

The Moment of Truth

Anticipating and visualizing are two important components in enabling you to succeed in this program. Another aspect is good old-fashioned positive thinking. Whether you are going to bed later at night or setting your alarm back in the morning, you will still have to deal with that difficult moment when the alarm goes off and you have to throw off the covers and jump out of bed before you drift off again. If you are like me, this is where you need a "crutch" or two to get you going.

Mental Crutches

Your first and most important crutch is the benefits we just discussed. By getting out of bed, you will take a step toward improving your life. You will be using time for the things you want to do, not what others want.

Next, I suggest you find a phrase that you can repeat to yourself in that semiconscious moment when your body rebels at the notion of getting up. No matter how motivated you are, I can guarantee you that there will be times when your alarm goes off, you moan, and the next thing you know, your 30 minutes has been traded for unconsciousness.

You need to program yourself to use a simple phrase to block out the excuses that your mind will use to preserve the comfort of your body. Find a phrase that is positive, motivational, and simple, such as these from Dr. Robert H. Schuller: "If it's going to be, it's up to me." "Inch by inch, anything's a cinch." Or tell yourself simply, "I can do it!"

I'm fond of a phrase from one of my son's storybooks, *The Little Engine That Could:* "I think I can, I think I can." When the alarm goes off, I immediately block out any negative thoughts with this chant. It sounds basic, I know, but without it my mind fills quickly with all the reasons why it is too cold to get up, how I can sleep just 10 minutes longer and still get everything done, why I deserve more sleep, or why I should skip my routine "just for today."

Physical Crutches

You can also use physical backups to make sure you get out of bed. Some people place their alarm clocks on the other side of the room so that they will have to get up to turn it off. Unless you sleep alone, however, I don't recommend this method. I think the negative feedback from a spouse could outweigh any of the positives of getting you up.

Instead, I recommend that you develop what I call a focal point. Pregnant women learn about focal points in childbirth class as a place or object to focus on to help take their minds off the pain of labor. In this case, the focal point helps take your mind off of the pain of getting out of your warm, snug bed.

Suggested Focal Points

¥ the coffeepot in the kitchen
¥ your running shoes by the front door
¥ an inviting chair in the living room
¥ the table on the patio
¥ the shower
¥ an exercise bicycle
¥ your television, ready to be turned on to an exercise show or tape

---

Your focal point should be specific. It should be in another room of the house. And it should be something that has either positive connotations (such as the coffeepot—if you are a coffee lover), or is so overwhelmingly motivating that you can't ignore it (such as your dog, scratching urgently at the door to go out).

You may have to experiment with choosing a focal point. I started with using my exercise bicycle as my focal point, but it was not a totally positive image for me at first. So I used a little one-cup coffee maker, which I placed in the guest bathroom. The first few days of the program I would turn off my alarm and repeat, "I think I can, I think I can" a dozen times as I walked zombielike to the coffee maker. As I pushed the little red button and began to smell the aroma of the coffee, I would be awake enough to avoid any temptation of returning to bed.

After I had been on the program for a while, I didn't need such a strong, positive focal point, so I returned to my exercise bicycle as motivator.

The Next Step

Eventually you may want to increase your bonus time. To have sufficient motivation, you will probably want to go beyond the immediate, short-term goals for using your time and add some long-term goals.

To develop long-term goals, start out by thinking big.
Ask yourself these questions:

1. What talents do I have that I've never really explored?

    _____

2. What interests do I have that I'd like to pursue?

    _____

3. What subjects in school interested me, but have long
    been forgotten?

    _____

4. If I could start my education and training over again,
    what other courses would I pursue?

    _____

5. What famous person would I be if I could be anyone—
    past or present?

    _____

6. When I close my eyes and picture the ideal setting for me,
    where am I?

    _____

If you'd like to do more brainstorming, try reading one of the
following books: *A Whack on the Side of the Head,* by Roger von
Oech; *Wishcraft,* by Barbara Sher; or *What Color Is Your Parachute?,*
by Richard Bolles.

Go ahead, let yourself dream. I know of a very successful
lawyer who uses his bonus time to pursue his love of art. Some
people know him as a partner in a major law firm; others know
him as an artist. He sleeps 4 hours a night and has been able to
successfully pursue two careers.

I know a woman who is an unassuming secretary during the
day. But during her extra time she has trained and run mara-
thons. She sleeps 5 to 6 hours each night.

So you've finally admitted it. You always wanted to be a ballerina or a race car driver or a professional tennis player. What does this have to do with sleep? Simple. Go back to your time pie and block out a small slice—15 minutes per day—for your dream. Now spend some more time brainstorming:

How could I spend fifteen minutes each day
to move closer to my goal?

In the next chapter you will learn how to specifically gain between 30 minutes and 2 hours extra each day. How much extra time you want will depend on how much you can actually use. Even before you start your program, begin to keep a wish list of your long-term goals, those dreams and crazy, secret ambitions, that you thought you'd never be able to pursue. Imagine what life will be like when you have the time to devote to those dreams!

SLEEPFACT: Babies in their mothers' wombs go through all the stages of sleep. Some research indicates that they even dream—although no one knows what they dream about.

Chapter Six

Step 3: Organization

Love not sleep, lest you come to poverty; open your eyes and
you will have plenty of bread.
—Proverbs 20:13

One of my favorite advertising slogans of all time is the one
used in a campaign for Nike running shoes: Just do it. If you are
at least curious about what you might do with extra time every
day, if you recognize some of the benefits of time for you, if you
are even mildly motivated, you are ready to *just do it!* There's no
way to explain more about the benefits of the sleep management
plan without letting you experience them for yourself.

We know that loss of sleep won't cause long-term physical or
psychological problems. In fact, we've seen how sleep reduction
actually helps some people. We've learned that the factors that
cause fatigue are often unrelated to sleep (or lack of it), and we've
discussed the need for more time to bring a sense of balance to
life.

Now it's time to really launch into the sleep plan and apply it
in your own life. This chapter·will give you the tools you need to
reduce your sleep and add hours to your life.

Your Sleep Log

I found it helpful to have a small notebook (I used a steno pad)
to use in managing my sleep. You may want to write your goals
for your extra time on the first page of your notebook. This will
be an easy way to reactivate your motivation.

Somewhere in the notebook you will want to start a sleep log, such as the one that appears on page 79. Copy it, or use it as a basis to create your own log. Whatever works for you is fine, as long as you can record your exact time into bed and out of bed. I tried both a log and a "sleep calendar" (pictured on page 80) and found that the calendar was more helpful for me, since I was used to planning my days and noting appointments on a calendar. I simply duplicated each month and used one calendar for my sleep log and the other for the rest of my daily appointments and reminders.

Begin to keep a sleep log before you begin to reduce your sleep. This is an important step that you might be tempted to skip. But just as the time pie showed where your time was going now, the sleep log will help you analyze how consistent you really are. Each day, for at least an entire week, record the time you go to bed, turn off the lights, and actually attempt to go to sleep. Then record the exact time the next morning when you first awaken. If you lay in bed for a few minutes and do not go back to sleep, that time is still your wake-up time. But if you fall back to sleep for more than 5 minutes, note that second time as well.

Don't feel any pressure during this week. Try to act as normally as possible and simply record these times without any sense of guilt. Be sure to note the times on weekends, too.

You may find yourself saying, "But this was an unusual week." If that's so, just record another week. I actually recorded an entire month *before I started* reducing my sleep because I kept telling myself that it had been an unusually erratic time in my life. When I analyzed that month I honestly had to say that my life was probably going to be like that for the next year or two, so I might as well get used to it.

Take a look at your recorded times after a week or two and note:

- How consistent is your bedtime?
- How consistent is your wake up time?
- How far do you deviate on weekends?

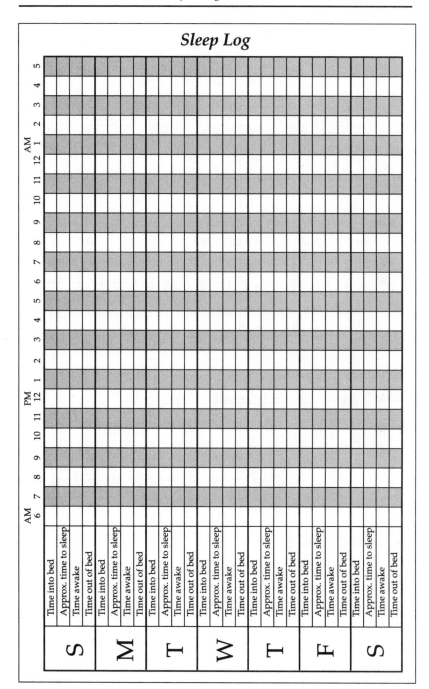

Sleep Log

Calendar

SUNDAY	MONDAY	TUESDAY	WEDNESDAY	THURSDAY	FRIDAY	SATURDAY
	7:00　　1 11:00	6:30　2 Start plan 11:00	6:30　3 11:30	6:30　4 11:00	6:30　5 11:30	7:30　6 12:30
8:00　7 11:00	7:00　8 11:15	6:30　9 11:00	6:30　10 11:30	5:00　11 ——— 10:00	6:00　12 L.A. → 10:30	13
14 ———————→	15	16	17	18	19	20
21	22	23	24	25	26	27
28	29	30	31			

Next ask yourself:

- What elements do I control?
- What elements don't I control?

You probably control the fact that you end up watching the late news each night, or that you like to watch Johnny Carson's opening monologue. You may not have much control over the time your spouse goes to bed or awakens.

Organizing Your Environment

One of the greatest surprises of the sleep management plan for me was realizing how much control I actually had over my environment. I had begun to feel that I was living my life at the whim of family, friends, and work. But when I began to analyze it, I found many ways to organize and control my life.

My greatest concern about starting to reduce my sleep was that I would awaken my husband if I got up early. I had to find a way to wake up and then quietly go about my routine without rousing him. I decided to turn our guest room into my early-morning room. I put an exercise bicycle in the room and moved in a small television set to use as I watched the early morning news show. I moved some of my toiletries into the children's bathroom to use for my morning shower. This all worked out surprisingly well. And after a few days of my early awakenings, Tom didn't even notice the alarm going off.

I was also somewhat concerned about running in the early mornings when it was still dark. I decided to exercise indoors on my bicycle from late fall through early spring, then take up running or walking during the spring, summer, and early fall mornings when the sun was up. Soon I discovered, however, that I could run along a major street early in the morning. I felt safe because of the lights, and had little threat from traffic since there were relatively few cars out. I had an option that I hadn't even considered!

Deciding on a Target Date

In the last chapter we discussed setting a target date for beginning the sleep plan as a way to increase anticipation and ensure motivation. The date you pick can have a great impact on how successful you will be.

For example, I first chose January 5 as my target date. It was at the beginning of the year, when my New Year's resolutions were still fresh in mind. It was long enough after the holidays to allow some time for recuperation. My older son was back in school and my husband and I had returned to our normal work hours. It seemed to make sense, but it was a total disaster for me.

There were two problems I had not counted on. The first was that I am a person who is very influenced by Seasonal Affective Disorder. January is one of the darkest months of the year where I live, and the lack of light was causing me to want to eat, sleep, and hibernate.

The second problem was the temperature. January and February are the coldest months in my area. I turn up my electric blanket each night before I go to bed and the difference between the air temperature in our bedroom in the morning and the temperature in my nice, warm, cozy bed is at least 10 degrees.

If you are sensitive to either light or temperature, you might want to check the averages for your area during the time you are targeting for your start date. I've included in the Appendix a chart of sunrise and sunset times for two latitudes because this turned out to be very helpful for me. Once I discovered that the sun rises in my area at approximately 6:30 A.M. on March 1, I targeted that as my start-up date. *Why not have the sun on my side?* I reasoned. The temperature also began to be on my side by March, giving me one less obstacle to overcome.

I have a friend who has just the opposite reactions to the seasons. She loves the short, cold days of winter and finds herself enormously productive from November through February. By the time the days lengthen and the temperature rises she is ready to go into summer hibernation.

You may be the type of person who has little or no reaction to these changes, or you may live in a place like Los Angeles, where the cold winds of winter rarely blow. If so, you can reasonably expect good results from almost any start-up time. But if you are like me—or my friend—be smart and choose a season that gives you a natural advantage.

Another important aspect of your start-up date is the day of the week. It was natural for me to think of Monday as a day to begin the new program. But I, like most people, had an even more erratic schedule on weekends, so getting up at my regular time was enough of a challenge on Mondays. Instead I chose a not-very-hectic Wednesday to launch my sleep management plan.

Setting the Goal

After looking at your sleep log and thinking through your lifestyle, it's time to decide where your extra time will come from.

You already have some idea as to whether you are an owl or a lark. But think about your environment as well. I know one two-career couple who decided that time together and time with their infant son were their two highest priorities. Since they both worked late—until about 7 P.M.—they were always feeling rushed in the evenings and barely had time with their son before his bedtime. They came up with the novel approach of putting their son on a new schedule with a bedtime of 11 P.M. That way they had plenty of time to play with him after work, he slept in the mornings while they were at work (a babysitter came to their home), and they would stay up until midnight to have some time alone with each other. They were actually able to sleep later in the mornings because they didn't have to deal with the baby as they were trying to run out the door. Both of them would have considered themselves "morning people," but the movement of their bedtime (and their son's) made more sense in their environment.

I am a lark married to an owl. When I started the sleep plan it was natural for me to get up earlier in the morning. But as I adjusted to my newfound time I decided to shave time off of my bedtime as well as my waking time. I didn't do this until my new waking time was firmly established, but in the end I was going to bed 30 minutes later, which made my husband happy, and waking up earlier, which made me happy.

Either your bedtime or your waking time should be fairly consistent.

The important principle to remember is that *either your bedtime or your waking time should be fairly consistent.* You are then able to manipulate the other time with a minimal amount of adjustment. If you have decided to commit yourself to waking up 30 minutes earlier in the morning, you must also commit yourself to a regular bedtime. It is more important that you be consistent in your sleep patterns than that you get a certain amount of sleep. That means that if you generally go to bed at 11 P.M. and get up at 7 A.M., you will probably feel better if you go to bed at the same time and get up 30 minutes earlier than if you go to bed two hours later and wake up two hours later.

Doing It . . .

One of the important elements of waking up the next morning, whether you are awakening earlier or have stayed up later, is setting your alarm. You really need to set two alarms: the alarm clock you keep by your bed and the one you keep in your head. The first is there to signal the time you should get up, the second is there to motivate you out of bed.

We talked about motivation in the last chapter. By now you should have many reasons for sleeping less. But you also need to *see* yourself rising out of bed, well rested, energetic and eager to begin your first activity. After you set your alarm clock at night, take a moment to lie back, close your eyes, and set your mind clock. Picture the time your alarm will go off in the morning. I have a digital clock radio, so I see digits; if you have a regular clock, picture the face with the hands pointed at your wake-up time.

In your mind, hear the alarm go off and see yourself simply reach over, turn off the alarm, and with one more motion sweep off the covers and step confidently out of bed. Then watch yourself move toward your focal point without looking back.

This may sound a bit contrived, but it makes an enormous difference in your ability to get up in the morning. I discovered this because periodically I must awaken at 4:30 A.M. to catch a very early flight. I discovered that I would anticipate the need for my wake-up time and would often open my eyes exactly at 4:29 A.M. so I could turn off the alarm before it awakened my husband. I didn't feel as if I had awakened abruptly, and I found that I rarely lingered in bed, since I knew how little time I had to dress and get to the airport. This made me aware of the enormous power of the subconscious (or unconscious) mind.

As I studied more about sleep patterns I was astounded by how much was a mental function and how little was physical. Our need for sleep, our perception of feeling rested, and our view of the quality of sleep we get are mostly a function of the mind, not the body. If we can harness that mind power it can be very helpful to us as we control and manipulate our sleep patterns.

Our need for sleep . . . is mostly a function of the mind, not the body.

You will also need to prepare your environment. Do as much preparation as you can the night before. Everything you need for your first 30 minutes should be out and ready. That includes your focal point. In warm weather I like to run, so I have my clothes and shoes sitting out in my bathroom where I can get dressed without disturbing my husband. I have my Walkman™ by the front door so I can grab it on the way out. If I am riding my exercise bicycle in the winter, I have the coffeepot ready to be switched on. I don't want to be fumbling with coffee grounds and water in my first few minutes of consciousness.

Make your preparation for the next morning part of your psychological warm-up for awakening. Be good to yourself. Prepare your environment so that everything is easy, available, and pleasant.

Establish a Schedule

We will talk more about the specific phases of sleep reduction in the next chapter, but in each phase you will need to prepare a schedule for the use of your time.

Use your notebook to write down your proposed schedule and then "image" it as you spend the moment setting your mental clock. I mentally watched myself go through my routine before I ever physically did it. I anticipated how good I would feel after exercise. I reaffirmed that prayer and Bible study would give me the right outlook on my day. I imagined waking up my children and husband gently, since I would feel under control and less hassled in the morning.

The additional 30 minutes I gained in the first phase of the sleep management plan had a significant impact on several areas of my life. And by sticking to my schedule, these beneficial activities became good habits in my life.

Don't be afraid to make adjustments to your schedule as necessary. You will probably want to accommodate the temperature and light changes depending on where you live. You will probably change your schedule completely as you add more time to your day. You may need to ease back into the program after an illness or vacation. Whatever the case, *write it down*. Make your schedule official.

Besides helping keep me committed to my program, my tools of organization helped me deal with the other people in my life. My husband took me more seriously as he watched me note my sleeping schedule. A friend at work decided that she would get herself organized just enough to see if the sleep plan was for her. After starting a notebook and mapping out her current schedule, she slid into the sleep plan with relative ease.

Take these steps to organizing your own sleep program today. You don't need to make a major commitment. But by finding out where you are and what you could do with extra time, you will begin to open a window to a whole new world.

SLEEPFACT: Napoleon went to bed between 10 P.M. and midnight, slept until 2 A.M., worked until 5 A.M., then slept again until 7 A.M.

Chapter Seven

Step 4: Patterning

We are all pilgrims and wayfarers in this life.
Arise then, pilgrim, shake off sleep for this is not the hour
for sleeping.

—Catherine of Siena

"Well, I tried your sleep management plan last week," Joanne announced, as we walked into a meeting together. I tried to remember what I had told her about my own sleep reduction. I could only recall a casual conversation in which Joanne had grown very excited when I told her I had reduced my sleep by 2 hours a night. But we'd never discussed how I had done it, and I wondered what Joanne meant when she said she'd tried the plan. My worst fears were soon confirmed.

"I had a big deadline and I knew I couldn't get everything done," she explained. "So I started getting up 2 hours earlier every day and going to the office before everyone else got in. It worked great for about 4 days. I made my deadline, and then I crashed. I went to bed on Friday night and woke up at noon on Saturday."

I groaned. "Joanne, that's not exactly what I meant by managing your sleep," I said. But then I realized I shouldn't be surprised when I thought about her pattern of food dieting. Joanne was a compulsive crash dieter. She regularly came into the office and announced that she had to lose 5 pounds by the weekend. She was an expert on every week-long diet, from liquid protein to grapefruits.

If you are a crash food dieter, like Joanne, you might be tempted to jump into sleep dieting with big goals and expectations for fast results. You may even find some limited success. A crash diet *can* take off 5 pounds in as many days. But a crash diet is not going to improve your lifelong eating patterns, any more than quickly cutting back your sleep is going to give you a balanced life-style. And the goal of sleep management is not so much to reduce sleep as it is to help you achieve balance in your life.

Before you decide to start the sleep management plan, commit yourself to one month of systematic sleep reduction. In that month you will gain at least 15 extra waking hours—an entire day you didn't have the month before. But, more important, you will gain a sense of control and balance. Instead of wanting to "crash" like my friend Joanne, you will be renewed and invigorated—and ready to go on to the next phase of the plan if you wish.

Phase I

Just the idea of having an extra 30 minutes in each day makes many people imagine what life would be like with 1 or 2 extra hours.

Adding as much as 2 extra hours to each day is within the range of many people. But the ability to get to that point and use that time happily and productively depends to a great degree on patterns you set in the first phase of the sleep management plan.

That is why proper patterning in the first phase of sleep reduction is so important. It allows you to give your body the right signals about sleep. Instead of feeling deprived, your system will begin to thrive on less sleep. Instead of fighting for sleep, your body will welcome the absence of fatigue. Instead of feeling down and gloomy, you will begin to feel a surge of mental energy.

With a good start, and depending on other circumstances in your life, you will be able to move on to Phase II within three weeks. Or you may choose to stay in Phase I, gratefully accepting the bounty of an extra 30 minutes a day.

Before you begin Phase I, you should have:
- a sleep log (see page 79)
- a start-up date (see pages 73, 81)
- short-term goals (see page 69)
- a proposed 30-minute schedule (see page 85)
- a focal point (see page 74)
- a positive phrase to repeat (see page 73)

Let's assume you have chosen a Wednesday in March for your starting point. Perhaps, as an extra incentive, you have made a date with a neighbor to meet you so that you can run together at 6:30 A.M. The night before you lay out your shoes and running clothes. You set your alarm back by 30 minutes. You note your bedtime in your sleep log, then spend about 30 seconds imagining yourself the next morning—bouncing out of bed, quietly dressing, then running out the door. You see yourself later in the day feeling energetic and healthy. You feel good about yourself, because you are taking a positive step toward gaining balance in your life.

The next morning you may have an experience like mine: I opened my eyes at 6:25 A.M., just minutes before my alarm was to go off. I pushed the button, bounded out of bed, and didn't even need my positive phrase to keep me going. I was at my focal point in 30 seconds flat and never looked back. *Wow! This is easy,* I told myself.

Bouyed by excitement, my first day was relatively easy. But my second and third days were harder. I was surprised by the noise of my alarm, and needed to repeat my phrase over and over again to block out the subliminal voice begging, "Just 5 more minutes."

My fourth and fifth days hit during the weekend and it took all my strength to get up at 6:30 on a Saturday morning. I knew it wouldn't be easy, so I planned a break from my routine and allowed myself a trip to a neighborhood coffee shop, where I read the paper and ate a roll.

Sunday I blew it. I shut off my alarm and the next thing I knew, I was awakening again to the sound of "Mommy, is it time to get up now?" My secondary alarm system woke me up at 7:15 A.M., a full 45 minutes later than my planned wake-up. I was frustrated that I'd fallen off the wagon, but was determined to get back into the routine.

Monday morning, the sixth day, I awakened at 6:25, once again before my alarm went off. What had often been my worst morning of the week felt good. I had exercised, showered, and was feeling good about myself and my day before the rest of the family stirred.

You feel good about yourself because you are taking a positive step toward gaining balance in your life.

The rest of the week went well. I began to think of 6:30 A.M. as my normal wake-up time. By the end of my second week, I was feeling better than ever.

My experience may be yours as well. The initial excitement may get you through the first few days, then level off, leaving you feeling discouraged. This is the most difficult time, because your body has not yet established a new pattern and is still fighting for the old wake-up time.

Don't worry. I can tell you from my own experience and the experience of others that this is a typical part of reprogramming your mind and body. Perhaps you'll want to plan a reward for yourself at this point. After you've been on the sleep plan for 7 days, why not buy yourself a present? We typically reward ourselves for losing weight, so why not reward ourselves for staying on this new program?

Another boost for me at this point was to listen to a positive-thinking tape series. Every day on the way to work I listened to a tape by a different "achiever." Just having positive thinking reinforced helped me fight off any discouragement I felt. It also helped me begin to formulate some messages, which I told myself each day:

- "I really feel great today."
- "I don't need much sleep."
- "It's a great day and I'm glad I got off to such a good start."

I was surprised by the importance these messages played in my life. When people asked me how my sleep plan was going I could answer honestly, "Great. I never felt better."

I also found myself less interested in coffee. In the past I had shuffled into the office and relied on a couple of cups of coffee to get me going. But my earlier wake-up time and the addition of exercise to my day gave me more energy. By the time everyone else arrived at the office, I was already feeling as if my day was under control. And when I could tell myself, "I really don't feel sleepy," I didn't feel inclined to drink coffee constantly.

After 3 weeks of sleep reduction you should find that cutting back your sleep by 30 minutes has become a natural pattern. If you do not feel comfortable with it, ask yourself some questions:

Are there circumstances in my life causing my fatigue?

Are relationships, work, finances, or other commitments creating stress and wearing you down? How can you cope with these problems directly, rather than sleeping them away?

Is there a physical problem that may be undiagnosed?

Is a lingering cold wearing you down? Have you been tested recently for anemia? Do you suspect that you may have a serious physical problem? If so, see your doctor.

Are the goals I set for myself really important?

Perhaps your reasons for having extra time seemed important, but really aren't. Is there something you'd rather do with your time?

Do you want to be good to yourself?

Psychologists say many of us are more afraid to succeed than we are to fail. Is there some reason why you don't want to achieve balance in your life? Do you find some form of security in always being out of control? Are you afraid of taking responsibility for your life?

Are others in my life undermining my efforts?

Does your spouse complain about your new pattern? Do people at the office tease you? Remember that change is never comfortable to anyone and some people think that your efforts to improve your own life imply condemnation of them.

If any of these reasons are causing you problems, you can either deal with them directly or you can simply go off the plan and try it again at a different time. During my first attempts at the sleep plan I had a cold, then I spent a week in Los Angeles—a full 3 hours off my time zone. Naturally I had to abandon the program during these times. (Waking up at 6:30 A.M. at home is one thing; setting my alarm for 3:30 A.M. in L.A. was quite another!)

> *Psychologists say many of us are more afraid to succeed than we are to fail.*

Surprisingly, I found that the patterns I had begun were very easily resumed; and even after abandoning my program for a week, I could go back to the earlier wake-up time in a day or two. Part of the reason for this, I am convinced, is that I simply came to believe that it was "normal" for me to awaken at the earlier hour.

I also found that it is much easier for me to manage my sleep in the spring, summer, and early fall than in the winter. This is probably true of many people, whether or not they share my photosensitivity. In Scandinavian countries, for example, people

Sample Schedules for Extra Time

Phase I		Phase II	
		6:00	Awaken; walk, pray, meditate, prioritize
6:30	Awaken; ride bicycle, pray, meditate, prioritize	6:30-6:45	Write in journal
6:45—7:00	Shower	6:45—7:00	Shower
7:00	Awaken family	7:00	Awaken family

literally shift their sleeping patterns by hours when the sun shines nearly around the clock in the summer months.

"I change my schedule," says Halvard Kvamsdal, deputy mayor of Kirkenes, a small town in northeast Norway. "I sleep only 3 or 4 hours during the summer."[1]

If you are struggling with a wake-up time that is before sunup, you might invest in a light box and hook it up to a timer. This "light alarm" is a much gentler way to be awakened and may help you cope with the darkness outside your window.

Once you have incorporated the extra 30 minutes into your day you are ready to move on to Phase II.

Phase II

After 3 weeks of extra time built into each day, it's tempting to want to add even more time rapidly. But, after trial and error, I discovered that most people should approach the second phase of the sleep management plan with some caution. You want to build on early successes, not undermine them.

Phase II is 4 weeks long and consists of 2 parts. The first 2 weeks add 15 minutes to your day; the second 2 weeks add another 15 minutes.

Why not just cut back another 30 minutes? The answer has less to do with your ability to cut back your sleep than it does with your ability to use the extra time. In theory we can always find ways to use an extra 30 minutes. But in fact your use of the extra time has to be compelling enough to overcome your natural tendency to sleep.

Here's how I went wrong the first time I entered Phase II: I felt great, I was totally convinced that I had never needed as much sleep as I had been getting, so I set my alarm back by another 30 minutes to 6 A.M. I didn't do a new schedule because I had already imagined all the ways I could use the extra time. The first day of Phase II I went to my focal point (the coffeepot), then turned on the television to check out the early news. Instead of getting on my exercise bicycle as I had done before, I sat down and started watching the news. After all, I had an extra 30 minutes, so there was no need to hurry.

I finally got to my exercise routine, then jumped into the shower. I took some extra time to condition my hair, then spent a few extra minutes on makeup. By the time I looked at the clock again it was 7 A.M. I had managed to waste my extra time by stretching out my routine.

The next morning my debate with the alarm clock went like this: "Maybe I'll just sleep in until 6:30. It doesn't seem to make that much difference anyway." I clicked off the switch and was awakened by my husband's alarm at 7 A.M. I was now back to the starting point.

How could you spend 10 or 15 minutes each day to work toward a long-term goal?

Learn from my mistake and *don't skip the scheduling* of your extra time. If you add only 15 minutes at first, you'll feel more compelled to make them count. I highly recommend that you schedule an entirely new activity into your extra 15 minutes, something that is important to you.

Look back in your sleep notebook at some of the long-term goals you scheduled for yourself. How could you spend 10 or 15 minutes each day to work toward a long-term goal? Develop a

Sample Timeshifts for Four Phases

	Phase 1	Phase 2	Phase 3	Phase 4
To bed	11:00 P.M.	11:00 P.M.	11:00 P.M.	11:30 P.M.
Awaken	6:30 A.M.	6:00 A.M.	5:30 A.M.	5:30 A.M.

new schedule for making use of your extra 45 minutes each day. Live with it for a few days and then make any adjustments necessary.

After 2 weeks consider adding another 15 minutes to your day. Remember, this will now give you 1 extra hour each day, or 7 extra hours per week. You may want to rethink your time usage altogether at this point. For example, instead of spending 15 minutes on my stationery bicycle I now had time for a 30-minute walk, which I preferred. I would spend my first 15 minutes listening to tapes as I walked, and I used my second 15 minutes to pray, meditate, and prioritize my day.

By adding the 30 minutes in 15-minute increments I was much more able to absorb the time, appreciate it, and find new ways to use it for my benefit. If you do not need this crutch, go ahead and jump right in to the extra 30 minutes. But remember to keep your wake-up or bedtime consistent, and schedule that extra time so you don't waste it. And be sure to check your physical responsiveness. If you begin to feel drowsy or irritable, don't push yourself. Perhaps you should be content to live with the extra 30 minutes.

Phase III

In Phase III you will be adding a total of 1½ hours to each day— or 10½ hours to your week. You may do this in either 2 additional 15-minute increments or one additional 30-minute increment.

If exercise has not been a part of your routine up to this point, you'll probably need to add at least a 10-minute warm-up to succeed. As we discussed before, your circadian clock signals a temperature increase when it is time for you to awaken. If you are resetting this clock by 1½ hours per day, you probably need to give your body temperature a quick boost at your wake-up time. Try running in place for 10 minutes, or just do 50 jumping jacks to get yourself going.

If you make it to this point, congratulate yourself. Most people won't have the determination to cut back their sleep by this much. Even the people who could do it physically are hampered by the mental obstacles.

Once you cut back your sleep time by the additional 30 minutes, be sure to analyze how you are feeling. Do you feel tired at any point during the day? Do you drift off while watching a television show in the evening? You may be hitting your personal limit. In chapter 9 we will discuss napping as a way to supplement your nighttime sleep. You may be at the point where a regular nap is necessary if you are to continue sleeping as little as you are at night.

> ### *Once you cut back your sleep time by the additional 30 minutes, be sure to analyze how you are feeling.*

At this point it is also important to take a look at the total amount of sleep you are getting. I started the program while getting an average of 8 hours of sleep each night. But if you started at seven hours and are now down to 5½, you may be struggling more than I was at this phase. Unless you feel absolutely fine, I wouldn't recommend that you consider reducing your sleep below 5 total hours of sleep per night.

There are, of course, people who regularly get less sleep. But unless you are being carefully monitored, I would be concerned about potential side effects of too little sleep.

An extra 1½ hours in your day allows you to make some new choices about how to spend the time. You may want to alternate schedules, such as playing tennis on Tuesdays and Thursdays, while maintaining your personal program on other days.

You may also choose to give yourself an extra 30 minutes of sleep on weekends. By the time you have cut back this far, letting yourself "sleep in" will probably not throw you off the program too far.

You may also reconsider where the time comes from. For example, I moved my wake-up time up by 1 hour and used the time effectively. But then I found that I preferred to have an extra 30 minutes with my husband in the evenings, so I established a new bedtime. In total, I cut back 1½ hours in the morning and 30 minutes in the evening.

Phase IV

Cutting back your sleep by 2 hours a night might have seemed unthinkable 6 months ago, but at this point you are ready to see if another 30-minute reduction is helpful to you.

You may find that this phase is actually easier than previous reductions were. Although there is no scientific evidence to support it, I couldn't help wondering if I was simply getting in sync with one of my "peaks" in my sleep cycle when I cut back to 6 hours of sleep. I actually awakened more easily after 6 hours than after 7.

By this point I had fewer debates with my alarm clock, but I also noticed that I could easily doze off if I leaned back in a chair in the middle of the afternoon. I didn't notice feeling sleepy during the day, but if the opportunity presented itself, I could "drop off" quickly. This was quite a contrast to my previous pattern of never being able to sleep during the day.

I theorized that I was reaching my optimum sleep/wake balance. I noticed that if I did not exercise (such as during the time that a pulled leg muscle slowed me down) I would feel fatigued in the afternoon.

On the positive side, I found that I hardly ever experienced jet lag anymore. My regular trips to cities with time zones that varied from 1 to 3 hours from my own hardly caused a ripple in my sleep patterns. I was becoming a more efficient sleeper.

Today I not only enjoy the many benefits that the extra 2 hours afford me each day, but I also find that I sleep better than I did before. I fall asleep almost immediately, rarely awaken, and rarely experience that vague feeling of "not sleeping well."

You may experience this at whatever phase of the sleep program you decide to incorporate into your life. You may find that you can experience a cutback of 2 hours in the summer, but only 1 hour in the winter. You may find that in times of stress you return to sleeping more. Experiment with yourself and your sleep. Read chapter 9 and try new ways to improve the efficiency of your sleep. Read the next chapter and try the tips on diet and exercise.

It's your life. As you find ways to enjoy it more, come back and try further reductions. You may find, like me, that the less you sleep, the more you enjoy the time you have.

SLEEPFACT: Danielle Steel, mother of 9 children and author of more than thirty books, sleeps less than 5 hours each night.

Chapter Eight

Step 5: Diet and Exercise

That which we are, we are. And if we are ever to be
any better, now is the time to begin.
—Alfred Lord Tennyson

Sara, John, and Chuck spent the morning working on a major presentation for a new client. The meeting was scheduled for 2:30 P.M. and they wanted to be completely prepared to explain their new ad campaign. When lunchtime rolled around they were still working, so a secretary in their office offered to go to the fast-food restaurant downstairs.

"Just bring me a hamburger with fries," John said. "And I'd like a Diet Coke—and get me a brownie, too. I deserve it," he said.

Chuck took a ham and cheese on a kaiser roll with a cup of soup and a 7-Up. Sara, who had sworn off junk food, ordered a tuna sandwich on whole wheat bread and a glass of skim milk.

The presentation went well until the client suggested a break at 3:30. "I could really use a cup of coffee," Sara said. John went into the bathroom to splash water on his face. Chuck went to the vending machine and bought a candy bar. "This room is really stuffy," he said as he returned to the meeting.

Although all the advertising executives had worked to prepare for the meeting, none had been prepared for the effect their lunch would have on their afternoon performance.

John's lunch, high in fat and carbohydrates, had begun to drain him of energy almost as soon as he'd finished it. His Coke gave him a slight boost for about 30 minutes, then he began to feel groggy. The brownie also gave him a quick boost, then gave him a "carbohydrate crash" about 3 hours later.

Chuck's lunch wasn't much better. Although he didn't have the caffeine, he did have a sandwich high in fat from the ham, cheese, and mayonnaise. The energy that went to process the fat could have been better used for the presentation.

Sara's lunch, though apparently healthy, was causing problems of its own. Although she didn't know it, Sara was mildly allergic to wheat grains and would begin to feel sluggish after eating whole wheat bread. In addition, her tuna and milk both contained high levels of tryptophan, the amino acid that tends to act as a sedative. When she yawned during the meeting, she attributed her fatigue to staying up too late the night before. In fact, she was more affected by her lunch than by her loss of sleep.

Each of the advertising executives was experiencing classic signs of fatigue, but none realized that the carry-out lunch was the real culprit. In fact, most people who begin to feel tired during the middle of the afternoon blame it on lack of sleep or poor sleep the night before. Many of us undermine our energy by the foods we eat each day, then try to make up for our fatigue by getting more sleep at night. No wonder Aristotle thought our need for sleep was part of our digestive process!

> *Many of us undermine our energy by the foods we eat each day, then try to make up for our fatigue by getting more sleep at night.*

It is possible to reduce your sleep substantially without ever changing your eating patterns or adding exercise to your daily routine. But both diet and exercise should be major considerations when you decide how much sleep you want to omit and how serious you are about bringing your life into balance.

I'm not a nutritionist or a personal trainer. In fact, when I began my own sleep reduction program I was simply a somewhat overweight, stressed woman whose idea of improving my diet meant cutting down on second helpings. But in researching sleep I kept bumping into food and fitness advice that made sense. This was not the "How to lose 5 pounds in 2 days" advice I usually read. It was more about what one could *gain* from healthful eating and regular exercise.

Energy, endurance, clarity of mind, and improved self-image were some of the by-products I read about. If I could patent a pill that would give people all these, I would be a millionaire. Yet I discovered some basic principles that meant these qualities were well within my range if I made a few changes to my daily routine.

I can't separate these principles from the sleep management plan itself, because the extra time in my day gave me the ability to incorporate them into my life. And the more I included them, the less sleep I needed and the more energy I enjoyed. There's nothing earthshaking about these principles. They are basic, tested advice from some of the best nutritionists and exercise enthusiasts around. But they work.

Eating for Energy

Many fine books include complete diet plans to increase energy. Two of the best are *Never Be Tired Again!*, by Drs. Gardner and Beatty, and *High Energy*, by Dr. Rob Krakovitz. For the purposes of this chapter, I will simply distill some principles of eating that can help improve your diet no matter what your life-style.

Principle 1: Cut Down on Fats

We've all heard that the American diet is too high in fats, and many of us have tried halfheartedly to make some changes such as switching to margarine from butter and to lowfat milk from whole milk. But we have a long way to go.

True, we are getting better. During my childhood our typical Sunday routine went like this: After church we sat down to a meal that usually included a beef or pork roast with gravy, rolls with butter, a vegetable such as creamed corn, and a big dessert. No wonder we all took Sunday afternoon naps! A meal like that would make anyone fall asleep while his or her body fought to process all of that fat.

How to Calculate the Fat Content of Your Diet

1. Add up all the calories you consume in a day.
2. Add up the calories of fat (look up the foods in a nutrition guide).
3. Multiply the calories of fat by 9.
4. Divide the answer by total calories consumed.
5. Multiply that answer by 100.

You should aim for a daily goal of less than 30 percent, although some doctors suggest reducing fat to less than 25 percent.

Have you ever cleaned the roasting pan after it has been sitting around for a few hours? Have you skimmed off the top layer of homemade chicken soup after it has been refrigerated? Then you know what fat is like in its most basic form. It is sticky, dense, and tends to congeal. What it does in the pan is almost exactly what it does in your blood.

When fat enters your bloodstream it attaches itself to red blood cells, which are normally going about their business of carrying oxygen to the brain. Fat literally gums up the process, slowing down the cells, making them less efficient, sometimes even causing them to stick to one another. Instead of delivering that oxygen supply on schedule, they fall behind. You may yawn in an attempt to pull in more oxygen.

If you have consumed enough fat your body has no choice but to send an urgent message to the brain: Shut down some systems so we can catch up. Your brain tells you to relax, lie down ... fall asleep.

So why not eat a meal high in fat right before you go to bed and enjoy the effects of this natural sleep inducer? Because your body is hard at work processing those fats and may, in fact, disrupt your natural sleep cycle. Almost like a sleeping pill, a fatty meal will help put you to sleep; but then its very presence inhibits your ability to get quality sleep.

The fat you eat will literally begin to immobilize you within an hour of your meal. Although you might never consider drinking wine with lunch, the ham sandwich or the fried chicken you eat may "drug" you just as effectively, impairing your performance for the afternoon. And over time the fat deposits will begin to stick to artery walls, building up and possibly even shutting down the very pipeline for oxygen to your heart, muscles, and brain. Not only will fat sap your energy, it will endanger your life.

Principle 2: Cut Down on Sweets

If you have a sweet tooth, like me, you may be tempted to skip this advice. After all, you know that a candy bar can supply a quick boost of energy. The problem is what comes after that boost. The high level of sugar in your body causes the pancreas to produce insulin. At first this gives your cells the ability to use the extra sugar. But when so much sugar flows in so quickly, the cells become saturated, causing the excess sugar to go into storage as glycogen.

Your energy level surges quickly, then falls below its former state. Your body relays a signal to the brain: Send down more sugar *now!* If you are within range of more M & M's you are likely to find your hand dipping into the candy dish almost without thinking. But if you have run out of your sugar source, or if your self-discipline takes over, your body rebels. Your blood sugar level drops. You may feel irritable, lightheaded, or get a headache. You will almost certainly feel tired.

Some people are hypoglycemic or have chronically low blood sugar. This occurs when your body produces too much insulin in reaction to the introduction of sugar into your system. The insulin tries to drive the blood sugar level down. If you suspect you may be hypoglycemic, you should talk to your doctor about developing a special diet plan. Typical diets include several smaller meals during the day and restricting sugars, alcohol, and caffeine.

If you have a sweet tooth, beware of using sugar substitutes. Several studies have shown that regular use of sugar substitutes actually acts as an appetite and sugar stimulant. Although you might have been satisfied with 1 teaspoon of sugar in your coffee, one of those little blue or pink packets gives you the sweetener of 2 teaspoons. You increase your threshold for sweets and tend to want more of "the real thing." In addition, some doctors fear other side effects of artificial sweeteners, and believe that they contribute directly to fatigue.

> *Just as you learn to reduce your need for sleep,*
> *you can cut back on your need for sugar*
> *and sugar substitutes.*

Just as you learn to reduce your need for sleep, you can cut back on your need for sugar and sugar substitutes. Not only will this change help your waistline, but it will also give you more energy during all your waking hours.

Principle 3: Eat on a Regular Schedule

Everything we have learned about our circadian clock builds a case for regularity. Our bodies like to know what to expect, whether it is bedtime or mealtime. Besides, eating on a regular schedule gives us the opportunity to rest and refuel every few hours, thus breaking the stress cycle.

Most people operate comfortably on a 3-meals-a-day basis. But you might experiment with a 4- or 5-meals-a-day schedule. Having smaller meals at shorter intervals may help you maintain a higher energy level without falling back on unhealthy snacks or excessive caffeine.

In addition to eating on a regular schedule, try to apportion your calories so that you get 65 to 75 percent of them *before* dinner. Many of us do just the opposite, and our constant battle of the bulge is a monument to this unhealthy pattern. Consuming fewer calories in the evening means that we have to creatively cut back heavy fat and protein consumption during the last meal of the day. And that's not a bad idea no matter when we implement it.

Principle 4: Cut Out Caffeine and Alcohol

We have already discussed the negative effects these two substances have on our ability to fall asleep and to sleep soundly. But even when they don't impair nighttime sleep, they are 24-hour-a-day energy sappers.

Both alcohol and caffeine can rob your body of important nutrients. They also cause the excessive highs and lows that trigger energy loss and may make your body seek refuge in sleep.

If you find yourself drinking more than 2 glasses of alcohol a day, whether through routine or desire, try to cut back on your own. If you find it difficult, consult your doctor or an addiction program in your area. You are not necessarily an alcoholic because you can't cut back alcohol on your own. Just as some people need a program such as Weight Watchers in order to follow through on a diet, you may need some help to impose the self-discipline it takes to cut back any comfortable habit. And if you have fallen into the habit of having a drink to relax you before bedtime, remember that the trade-off may be poorer quality sleep at night.

Although I am still a believer in using coffee to "jump start" me in the mornings, I have learned to cut caffeine out of my diet during the rest of the day. A few years ago I spent a week at a health spa, where I hoped to lose some pounds and tone up some muscles. What I didn't expect was to discover that I was a caffeine addict. After a day and a half on the salt-free, caffeine-free diet, I suffered from headaches, dizziness, and serious fatigue. It had never occurred to me that my occasional trips to the office coffeepot, combined with my diet sodas, had added up to a whopping dose of caffeine each day. But going through with-drawal convinced me that I'd never allow myself to get hooked again.

I don't recommend going cold turkey. But if you suspect that you are drinking too much coffee, start mixing your regular grounds with decaffeinated in an increasing proportion. Or try the new instant coffee that has 50 percent less caffeine. Over a period of a month even the most hardcore addict should be able to cut down to less than 200 mg. of caffeine a day (approximately 2 cups of brewed coffee).

Principle 5: Beware of "Hidden" Sleep Agents
Three other types of foods can sap your energy and cause fatigue: foods to which you are allergic; those to which you have a certain sensitivity; and foods that contain substances such as tryptophan, which can increase drowsiness.

Food allergies are far more common than most of us realize. A friend of mine who consulted a nutritionist was shocked to discover that he was allergic to wheat products. Even as a child he had happily consumed Shredded Wheat for breakfast, never imagining that some of his inability to concentrate in school might have been tied to his "healthy breakfast." Food allergies can cause skin problems, migraine headaches, intestinal disturbances, and fatigue. They may even be responsible for dizziness, inability to concentrate, and arthritis.

The most common food allergies are to grains, dairy products, and fermented foods (including alcohol). You might try to eliminate all these from your diet for a period of three days, then reintroduce them one at a time for three days each. If you have a reaction, it will be more noticeable. You should also consult your doctor or a nutritionist, especially if your reactions are acute.

Food sensitivities may actually be food addictions. Some doctors believe that we become addicted to certain foods that are actually detrimental to our systems. The person who craves chocolate, for example, eats a piece and gets both a sugar and caffeine high. She then drops to a new low and craves more chocolate to bring her back up again.

If you crave any food, beware of the impact it is having on you. A friend of mine seemed to eat an amazing amount of yogurt,

---

Foods High in Tryptophan

Buttermilk	Lima beans	Parmesan cheese
Chicken	Liver	Peanut butter
Cottage cheese	Macaroni	Rice
Eggs	Milk	Tuna
Halibut	Nuts	
Ice cream	Oatmeal	

---

which didn't seem like a terribly unhealthy habit. That is, until she realized that the sugar content of the particular yogurt she was eating was higher than that of a candy bar! She was actually on a sugar high all day.

Another hidden energy sapper is any food that contains tryptophan. As we've already learned, this naturally occurring amino acid is a great sleep inducer. It is found in milk (probably accounting for the common wisdom that a glass of warm milk will help you sleep), tuna, peanuts, bananas, and other common foods (see the chart).

Principle 6: Drink Plenty of Water and Eat Lots of Vegetables and Complex Carbohydrates

Instead of thinking about all the things you can't eat, try to concentrate on all the great foods available to you. Learn to enjoy steamed vegetables. Take a tip from oriental cooking and learn how to use spices such as ginger and garlic to enhance the natural flavors of vegetables.

Concentrate on filling up your diet with complex carbohydrates, such as baked potatoes, pastas, and wild rice. Many are what we have learned to call "comfort foods," and apparently complex carbohydrates actually do soothe your body and offer it a great source of long-term energy. Instead of dowsing these foods with butter, use a butter substitute such as Molly McButter. I began serving this on foods for my finicky husband and even for guests, and so far no one has guessed that I'm not serving the real thing.

Water is a secret weapon that every dieter should use. Drinking 8 glasses a day may seem daunting, but try buying a 1.5-liter bottle of water and carrying it with you. I drink it while working at my desk, commuting in the car, and relaxing with a book. You can go through a bottle in a day without much trouble if you take a gulp every now and then. And you'll stave off hunger pangs. The best thing about water is that it eliminates waste from your system without flushing away essential vitamins and minerals as coffee or sweet drinks can. It's a natural way to add energy to each day.

Exercise

What is the safest, most effective energizer available without prescription? It doesn't have to cost a thing, it is available in various forms to anyone, and its side effects are completely safe. It is, of course, exercise, and no book that talks about a balanced life can overlook the importance of this element. Says Dr. Holly Atkinson, "It is safe to say that a woman who does not exercise regularly has some degree of chronic fatigue."[1]

My grandparents grew up on farms and eventually ran one of their own. Although I doubt either one of them ever jogged (except to catch a cow that had escaped from the pasture) or did sit-ups, daily exercise was a part of their lives. Until my grandfather died suddenly at 90 he still had more energy than most men half his age. His mind was sharp and his arms were muscular.

My father left the farm for the city and has sat behind a desk most of his life except for a weekly game of golf. And my life tended to be even more sedentary, except for occasional spurts of enthusiasm for health clubs.

The main reason I wanted to have more time was to work daily exercise into my routine. I believed it would help me lose weight and stay in shape. And in doing so I became a confirmed believer in the power of exercise to energize.

What's so good about exercise? First, it increases your metabolism—not just during your workout, but also for hours afterward. It helps your blood flow efficiently, your heart beat rapidly, and it even helps you eliminate waste through perspiration. Second, it helps eliminate stress by relieving tension and helping to release the body's own tranquilizers. And third, it burns calories, causing fat to be burned instead of clinging to artery walls and sugar to actually be used by the body instead of causing an insulin rush.

Exercise also elevates body temperature slightly, and, as we discussed in chapter 7, this can help awaken you naturally. It is also a good reason to *not* work out within 2 hours of your expected bedtime. The temperature increase and the natural high from exercising can send signals to your body such as "Wake up, get going, don't relax."

> ### *Exercise after work or before dinner is a good way to release the accumulated stress from the day.*

Regular exercise at any time is good for you. Most people, however, exercise first thing in the morning, after work, or before dinner in the early evening.

The advantage of early morning is that you probably have more control over your schedule then and can comfortably fit exercise into a daily routine. It can also start you off for the day with a boost of energy and positive mental reinforcement. (I always feel a little smug about finishing my exercise before most people awaken.)

Exercise after work or before dinner is a good way to release the accumulated stress from the day as well as to act as a natural appetite suppressant for the evening. If you have a problem controlling your appetite in the evenings you might find that 20 to 30 minutes of exercise at this time of day helps you reduce your calorie intake before bedtime.

What kind of exercise should you do? Many people get discouraged because they can't see themselves running 5 miles or

Caloric Usage of Various Activities Done
for 30 Minutes

ACTIVITY/EXERCISE	120-POUND WOMAN (calories)	160-POUND MAN (calories)
Badminton	180–220	220–260
Baseball	160–200	200–240
Basketball	300–400	400–600
Bicycling moderately	100–120	120–140
Bicycling energetically	200–230	280–320
Bowling	80–120	100–140
Canoeing	100–150	130–180
Climbing stairs	130–160	160–190
Dancing moderately	100–130	130–170
Dancing energetically, disco	200–400	250–500
Exercising moderately	140–170	180–220
Exercising energetically	200–250	250–350
Football	250–300	300–400
Golf, no cart	100–140	130–170
Handball	200–350	300–400
Horesback riding	140–160	160–200
Jogging, light	200–250	250–300
Lacrosse	250–350	350–400
Rowing vigorously	300–400	400–500
Running	300–400	400–500
Skating energetically	200–300	250–350
Skiing energetically	200–300	250–350
Soccer	250–350	350–400
Squash	180–240	250–400
Swimming steadily	200–300	300–400
Table tennis	150–180	200–250
Tennis, amateur	180–220	250–280
Volleyball	180–220	220–280
Walking moderately	80–100	90–120
Walking energetically	140–160	160–180

swimming laps in the pool each day. But many types of exercises offer aerobic (which simply means "utilizing oxygen") benefits. One of the most popular is walking. For more ideas read Dr. Kenneth Cooper's excellent book, *The Aerobics Program for Total Well-Being.*

As a reformed couch potato I can only offer you the advice that worked for me: Find an activity you like, do it daily (in moderation), and promise yourself you will stick with it for 6 weeks. My bet is that after that time you'll be hooked. And that's the kind of addiction that can add years to your life.

Without a regular exercise program you may not be able to move to the highest levels of the sleep plan. But if you cut out an additional 30 minutes of sleep and then devote much of that time to exercising, you can probably cut back your sleep even further. And, based on my own experience, the hours that you have available to you every day will be filled with less stress, more energy, and more peace of mind.

SLEEPFACT: Men over the age of 60 have no Stage 4 sleep at all. Women seem to experience more deep sleep as they get older.

Chapter Nine

Step 6: Efficient Sleep

He sleeps well who knows not that he sleeps ill.
—Publilius Syrus

Perhaps one of the greatest by-products of the sleep management plan is that it can lead to improving the quality of your sleep. This is not just an imagined benefit. Studies in sleep laboratories show that consistent sleep reduction causes a person to actually *increase* the amount of deep sleep in the first few hours of the sleeping period. It's as if the body tells the sleep mechanism, "No fooling around now. Go for the quality sleep right away."

Says Mayo Clinic's Dr. Hauri:

> What happens if you're a 7-hour sleeper and stay in bed 9 hours? . . . after several weeks, the 7 hours of sleep would get spread thinly over all 9 hours. It is as if a given amount of water were spread over a much larger surface, no longer covering it well. This shallow sleep is much less restorative, and you wake up more tired and weak than before.[1]

In fact, a study that measured the various stages of sleep in short-sleepers (6½ hours per night) and very-short-sleepers (5½ hours per night) discovered that both groups had as much or more deep sleep than the groups of sleepers who averaged 7½ or more hours of sleep per night. The difference came in Stage 1 sleep (sleep that is just barely removed from wakefulness) and Stage 2 sleep (slightly deeper, but not REM sleep). There was also a difference in REM sleep among the groups, but it was not as significant as the differences in Stage 1 or Stage 2 sleep. "Their sleep was less disturbed and more efficient," concludes Dr. Horne in his analysis of the short and very short sleepers.[2]

Once you have reduced your sleep you will probably notice that you go to sleep more quickly, sleep more soundly, and have fewer episodes of nighttime awakenings. As my husband observed, "You sleep like a log now."

It is true that I became a sounder sleeper after I reduced my sleep. But I also learned some important principles about sleep that I shared with my husband. Even without going on my sleep reduction plan, he learned to improve the quality of his sleep.

Many of these principles seem like common sense. But if you follow them carefully you should be able to further improve your sleep whether you reduce it or not.

1. Don't Spend Too Much Time in Bed

As basic as this sounds, sleep specialists have found that many insomniacs sit in bed for hours—reading, watching television, or lying awake and thinking. By restricting the time these people actually spend in bed, the specialists have helped them mentally and physically see bed as a place for sleep.

Another method that doctors use with those who can't sleep is to restrict their time in bed. If you have trouble falling asleep after more than 20 minutes, get up, go to another room of the house, and do something else. Don't allow yourself to go back to bed until you are absolutely exhausted.

Don't fret about not getting enough sleep. We have already learned that lack of sleep doesn't do any serious damage to your mind or body, that you should be able to perform even complex tasks with little or no sleep, and that you can make up for your lack of sleep by getting approximately 25 percent more sleep tomorrow night. Just reminding yourself of some of these facts can take the pressure off.

If you consistently lie awake at night for more than 20 minutes, begin to reduce your sleep by an additional 30 minutes. You may have not yet arrived at your optimum amount of sleep and are still sleeping too long. Many of the people who think they are insomniacs are simply naturally short sleepers. You may need even less sleep than you think.

2. Establish a Regular Schedule

We have already discussed the need for consistency as part of the sleep plan. But even when you are not reducing sleep you are sending signals to your "sleepostat," telling it what to expect. If you go to bed at 11 P.M. every night, then start staying up until 1 A.M., your body will begin to adjust, believing that it is being trained for a new bedtime. This is why so many people have a hard time getting to sleep at their "regular" time on Sunday nights after staying up later on Friday and Saturday. Their body has readjusted to a new time and needs a day or two to switch back.

An hour or two before your established bedtime, your body temperature begins to fall, your system slows down, and you begin to relax. If you were being monitored in a sleep lab, there would be evidence of slowed brain activity. Just as you begin to feel hungry around your normal lunch time, your body sends signals to your brain that bedtime is approaching. It begins to make the gentle transition toward sleep before you get into bed.

Be good to yourself and go to bed at the same time each night.

But if you change your bedtime regularly, your sleepostat goes haywire. It gets confused signals. Your brain learns that it better not relax since it might be called upon to party. Your body temperature begins to fall and your brain overrules it, using precious energy to fight itself. A debate of sorts goes on among your systems:

"I'm sure it's time to start shutting down."

"Not yet. Remember how we all relaxed last night at this time, then she went out dancing and it took a while to get back up to speed."

"Let's stay prepared just in case. We have to be ready if we're needed."

If you've ever changed time zones, you know how your body feels when it is expected to go out to dinner just when it would normally be going to bed. You can almost feel the debate raging. Hunger pangs are forgotten as the desire for sleep takes over.

Be good to yourself and go to bed at the same time each night. If you have tried the sleep plan and have established a new wake-up time or bedtime, stick to it—even on weekends. Over the long run you will find it easier to maintain a shorter sleep time if you don't send mixed signals to your sleepostat. In fact, you will feel better and sleep better if you settle into a regular pattern of sleeping and waking hours.

3. Prepare the Environment

How many times have you gone to bed only to get up again a few minutes later to adjust the thermostat, close a window, or turn off a light? Even when we are near exhaustion, some distraction in our environment can keep us awake or awaken us out of a deep sleep.

Go through a quick checklist before going to bed. Is the temperature in the room comfortable? Will it be too cold by morning if you leave the window open? Are the lights out and is the room darkened properly to guard against early morning light?

Is the bed itself comfortable? My husband can't stand "scratchy" sheets and will toss and turn if the linens are too crisp. I, on the other hand, will lose sleep if I stay in a hotel that provides a very fat pillow. Beware, too, of down pillows and comforters if you have allergies. You may sniffle and sneeze all night, never realizing that your nose is buried in the very source of your reactions.

Is there a cover nearby in case you get cold in the night? Our body temperature drops when we sleep and even on a warm summer night we can experience a chill in the early morning hours. There's nothing more maddening than trying to stay warm and having our sleep constantly interrupted by the shivers.

4. Establish a Bedtime Routine

Most of us have bedtime routines whether we notice them or not. We check to see that the doors are locked, the kids are tucked in, and the lights are turned out. But some sleep specialists suggest extending the routine to as much as 1 hour before bedtime to begin to clue your body to slow down.

A glass of milk is a good relaxer if you have a hard time drifting off. You might sit and read quietly for an hour before bed. A warm bath is another soothing routine that can signal bedtime.

Don't get into the habit of exercising before bed, which will raise your body temperature and stimulate your senses. And don't watch the late news if it tends to upset you and cause you to worry.

Don't get into the habit of exercising before bed.

Some people like to listen to classical music as they fall asleep. Others have learned to depend on a tape recording of falling rain, waves lapping on a beach, or wind rustling in trees. As simplistic as it seems, the cue you get from these sounds will help signal your body to slow down and relax.

You might also practice relaxation exercises or learn biofeedback exercises, which can help relieve stress. Tests show that people who are relaxing with such methods actually have brain activity that is similar to the early phases of sleep.

5. Don't Take Your Worries to Bed

I have heard people recommend that you "sleep on a problem"—that is, you think about it just before you go to bed and by morning a solution may come to you subconsciously. Maybe this method works for some people, but when I've tried it I've ended up lying awake for hours, then falling asleep and having nightmares about the problem. I try to not think about *any* problems before bedtime.

There's nothing worse than developing a nighttime worry habit. It's probably the cause of most of sleep problems in this country. Some people even come to associate bedtime with worries. After a relatively calm day, they lie down for the night and pull out all their concerns to chew on for minutes or hours.

There's nothing worse than developing a nighttime worry habit.

Some people even worry about not sleeping. Just remember, not sleeping won't kill you, but worry can. It will deplete your energy, give you ulcers, undermine your self-confidence, and interfere with your immune system. If you have any tendency to worry, read Dale Carnegie's *How to Stop Worrying and Start Living.* It could add years to your life.

If you have a tendency to worry about forgetting something you have to do the next day, make it part of your bedtime routine to write your to-do list for the next day. Once you have completed the list, *forget about it.* Don't lie in bed trying to remember if there is anything you forgot to add.

If you tend to lie in bed and feel anger or hatred or remember the ways people have wronged you, remember that they are the winners if they can also rob you of sleep and peace of mind. One simple solution I have found for dealing with frustrations I have with others is to pray for them. I tell God that I'm angry and frustrated. Then I ask him to help me be open to the person, to understand where he or she is coming from, to take my anger away, and to help me forgive the person. It is very difficult to hold onto anger or hurt when you have prayed for the person. Time and time again, I have awakened with a remarkably calm attitude toward the person who caused me so much anxiety just the day before. Several times I've actually had someone apologize to me. But mostly, I have learned that peace is something worth fighting for and I refuse to go to bed with anger or worry dominating my mind.

6. Eat Enough, But Not Too Much

Hunger pangs can keep you awake even when your mind and body crave sleep. If it's helpful, have a snack of cookies and milk an hour before bedtime.

Don't eat a heavy meal too close to bedtime. Even though we have seen how sugars or fats will make you sleepy, your body will also be spending a great deal of energy on digestion which can disrupt your sleep.

Become aware of foods that seem to interrupt your sleep. I have learned that a Chinese meal made with monosodium glutamate (MSG) or heavy doses of soy makes me sleep poorly and I often awaken with a slightly swollen face. Now that I eat little red meat I find that a steak dinner leaves me feeling as if I have a brick in my stomach at bedtime.

Beware, too, of spicy meals that taste great going down, but upset your stomach just as you turn in for the night.

You don't have to become excessively concerned about everything you eat, but remember that what you eat at dinner may have an effect on how readily you fall asleep a few hours later.

7. Avoid Alcohol and Caffeine Before Bedtime

Only you know how long before bedtime you can drink a cup of coffee without lying awake for hours. I have a 5 P.M. rule: I drink no coffee or colas nor do I eat chocolate after this time. I also have learned to avoid medications that include caffeine, such as Excedrin. (See chapter 2 for a complete list of medications containing caffeine.)

If you are having difficulty falling asleep, you should cut back on caffeine altogether, since its effects may be felt for hours after you consume it. And remember that there are several sources of caffeine in our diets, so don't just cut out coffee and think you've solved your problem.

I know that an evening glass of wine or other alcohol is a tradition with some people. If it helps you relax and you have good quality sleep, fine. But if your sleep is restless or disturbed, alcohol could easily be the culprit. Substitute a warm glass of milk or herbal tea for your alcohol, and you may find that your sleep improves dramatically.

> ### *If your sleep is restless or disturbed, alcohol could easily be the culprit.*

8. Exercise Regularly, But Not at Night

Can daily exercise improve sleep? Absolutely. People who exercise regularly tend to have longer periods of deep sleep, fall asleep more quickly, and have fewer sleep disturbances.

If you go out for the first time in months and run a few miles, this may not be the case. Your sore muscles may keep you awake despite the positive effects of the exercise. But, over time, regular aerobic exercise will act as a great aid in promoting efficient sleep. Your body will be processing oxygen more effectively, your systems will be "tuned up," and stress should decrease as your physical activity increases.

Exercise 1 or 2 hours before bedtime acts as a stimulant and tends to raise body temperature. If you are trying to stay up later, exercise is a good way to extend your waking hours and increase your concentration. But if you want to fall asleep rapidly, confine your exercise to morning, afternoon, or early evening.

9. Avoid Sleeping Pills

We have already discussed the problems with many sleep remedies. Although they may cause you to fall asleep, they can keep you from getting the deep sleep you need to feel rested. They may interfere with REM sleep and the ability to dream. They may even leave you with a "hangover," making you feel dizzy or disoriented.

If you have been taking sleeping pills regularly, especially the prescription type, you should wean yourself gently so you don't experience discomfort or side effects. Many sleeping pills are very strong narcotics, and you are likely to have some type of addiction if you have been taking them regularly.

10. Consider Adding Naps to Your Routine

The idea of taking out 60 minutes from our busy day to relax and sleep seems impossible to most of us. Yet in other cultures, a day without a siesta (or whatever it might be called) would be unthinkable. In Europe most shops close down completely between 1 P.M. and 3 P.M. Everyone goes home to enjoy the big meal of the day, to see their family, and to sleep.

There are very good reasons to take a nap in the middle of the afternoon. In many countries the temperatures peak at this point, causing outdoor work to slow. And our circadian cycle tends to go through one of its two low points in midafternoon (the other being around 3 A.M.). We lose our ability to concentrate, we often make mistakes at work, and some of us even yawn and put our heads down on our desks for a minute or two.

Many people in other countries use the nap as a way to shift some of their sleep time from night to day. In other words, they may sleep 1 hour in the afternoon and then 6 hours at night, giving them 7 hours of sleep for the 24-hour period.

There are many famous nappers in history. Winston Churchill said, "Nature had not intended mankind to work from eight in the morning until midnight without the refreshment of blessed

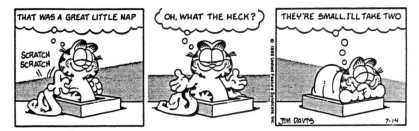

There are many famous nappers.

oblivion." Churchill enjoyed that oblivion almost daily. Napoleon was also a regular napper, managing to rest even in the middle of his most ambitious campaigns.

Thomas Edison napped and so did Mozart. Salvador Dali had an unusual way of napping: He sat in a chair, dangling a teaspoon between two fingers. The spoon was positioned over a metal plate. As soon as Dali fell asleep, the spoon would fall and awaken him with its clatter. This was his idea of enough sleep.

While mayor of New York, Ed Koch liked to sleep in his limousine between appointments (as he was stuck, no doubt, in Manhattan gridlock); and Ronald Reagan brought the art of napping to the public eye as he frequently nodded off at meetings.

So why should the rest of us nap? First, because our bodies want to sleep at midafternoon. Nearly all of us are less productive then than during other times of day. Second, napping allows our bodies a respite from stress and physical work, giving us a chance to bounce back and have a surge of productivity in late afternoon. And third, a daily nap gives us the ability to cut back our nightly sleep.

An occasional nap will probably only hurt your ability to sleep at night.

The key here is *regular* napping. An occasional nap will probably only hurt your ability to sleep at night. But a daily nap at a regular time will fit right into your daily cycle and won't have any negative impact on your nighttime sleep.

How do you work it out? Many people enjoy naps as one benefit of a home-based business. Others take a late lunch hour and relax in their office with the door closed. Many at-home mothers know that napping when their children do can give them a much better outlook for late afternoon and evening activities.

Some employers are even considering instituting a rest break, because productivity has been shown to be improved by as little as 20 minutes of rest during midafternoon.

> **SLEEPFACT: In 1983 a United States Circuit Court ruled that the right to sleep is protected by the First Amendment to the Constitution.**

Chapter Ten

Questions and Answers

I wake to sleep and take my waking slow. I learn
by going where I have to go.
—Theodore Roethke

My search for answers to my own questions about sleep made me the resident sleep expert among my friends. Over the months that I researched this book I was asked so many questions about the subject that I almost gave up my original idea for the book in favor of doing a book full of questions and answers.

During the course of my search I stumbled upon so many interesting facts about sleep and sleep-related matters that it seemed a shame to leave them out if they didn't relate directly to my subject. So I've tried to narrow the questions to those I was asked most frequently, or those that provide the most insight into the marvelous and sometimes mysterious subject of sleep.

I must say, once again, that I am not a doctor, researcher, or scientist. I am simply a person who became fascinated with sleep once I realized that many of my assumptions were false. The answers to most of these questions come from the many books and articles I have read on the subject. In some cases I have footnoted the answers to give the reader a source of more information.

Sleep and Work

Is it dangerous to change shifts? How long does it take to adjust?

Many studies are being done about the effects of shift changes on shift workers. More accidents occur when a worker has changed shifts within the last 72 hours, and a person's private life also suffers, often causing depression. The amount of time needed to adjust depends on the person and whether the shift was from day to night or night to day. Within 10 days most people are thoroughly adjusted to a complete shift change.

Charles Ceizler at Brigham and Women's Hospital in Boston has found that 39 percent of shift workers either have accidents or barely avoid them as a direct result of being sleepy at work. Twenty-nine percent reported automobile accidents related to sleepiness.

In *Wide Awake at 3:00 A.M.*, Richard Coleman says, "Asking the biological clock to adjust to new schedules, whether as a result of work shifts or of jet travel, can put a real strain on a system."[1]

I have to travel across time zones a great deal. How can I reduce jet lag?

Crossing time zones is very much like changing shifts. Your body gets external cues that are inconsistent with the internal clock by which it has learned to expect food and sleep.

The best way to fight jet lag is to anticipate the time change you will experience and begin to adjust a few days ahead of your trip. Begin to change your sleeping times as well as your meals, if possible.

You may also find, as I did, that reducing your sleep reduces your jet lag. When I slept 8 or more hours each night, I found it very difficult to adjust to a 3-hour time difference. Now, with my sleep reduced to 6½ hours, I rarely experience any problems with jet lag.

Sometimes work piles up and I end up getting much less sleep than normal for as much as a week. Is this dangerous?

Lack of sleep is not in itself dangerous. However, the amount of stress and tension related to work during a pressure time *is* dangerous and can sap your energy more than your lack of sleep will.

It is also better to cut back your sleeping hours gradually and stay somewhat consistent than to get 7 hours one night and 4 hours the next. If you anticipate a busy time at work, why not cut your sleeping time by 30 minutes to 1 hour before things get out of hand? You'll probably be more productive.

Also, if you need to cut back on sleep, do try to get at least 30 minutes of exercise each day, eat fewer fats, and minimize your caffeine intake (not below your normal level). These factors will help you feel more energetic and exercise will help you reduce the stress that can exaggerate fatigue.

While You Sleep . . .

Is it true that dreams are linked to memory?

Yes. Studies show that dreams are recapitulations of experience and can aid learning. When REM sleep is deprived, memory of new tasks is impaired, according to Dr. David Hawkins of Michael Reese Hospital in Chicago. "REM sleep and dreaming reflect a busy period of brain activity when new material is being processed," he says.

Dr. Hawkins also believes that dreams may be a link to the future. "We may attempt to play out in a dream, rather than in reality, what might happen if one course or another were undertaken."[2]

Should we be concerned about how much sleep a doctor has had before he treats us? I have heard that many residents in hospitals are sleep deprived.

Many medical residents work 80- to 104-hour weeks, often on 36- to 48-hour shifts. Although they may become irritable and may even suffer some short-term memory loss, studies show that they are just as capable as their well-rested counterparts of performing intricate tasks. Still, many states are considering legislation that would limit residents to 80-hour work weeks. Most doctors oppose the curtailing of residents' hours.

Can you learn new skills, such as a language, while asleep?

Yes. According to Dr. Robert Bjork of UCLA, studies show that learning can take place while a person is technically asleep. One study found that military recruits learned Morse code three weeks faster when they underwent sleep learning. However, sleep learning does interrupt normal sleep cycles and can interfere with a person's ability to feel well rested. The cost "might be justified under the right conditions," according to Bjork.[3]

Can you control the subject of your dreams?

Stephen La Berge of Stanford University believes you can. In his book *Lucid Dreaming* he discusses several exercises you can do to influence the content and length of your dreams. He also suggests that you may be able to influence your waking behavior by dreaming of yourself as you want to be. For example, if you are too shy, he suggests that you try to dream about yourself as outgoing.

Why do we feel sleepier when we are sick?

When the body is fighting a virus, it uses all its available energy very quickly. Your body has fewer energy requirements while asleep, thus giving your body the ability to devote more energy to helping you get well.

In addition, some scientists believe that certain bacteria actually trigger a sleep response in the brain. James Krueger of the University of Tennessee at Memphis says that normal bacteria may actually be the cue your brain gets in order to sleep. So when additional bacteria enter the system through illness, the brain gets more signals that sleep is needed.[4]

Is it a good idea to "sleep on a problem" in the hopes that it will be solved subconsciously while you are in bed?

Some people use this method regularly. But if you have any problems falling asleep or sleeping soundly, I'd discourage you from trying it.

If you would like to see if it works, simply pose your problem to yourself right before going to bed. When you awaken in the morning, write down the first ideas that come to mind. "Dreams are a natural problem-solving function of the mind," says Gayle Delaney, a psychologist and dream consultant in San Francisco.[5]

Her book *Living Your Dreams* has been used in a course at Stanford's Graduate School of Business and contains many ideas for using dreams to solve problems or create new opportunities.

How important are dreams to our mental health?

Freud thought dreams were the key to our subconscious mind and were very important to our health. But Nobel laureate Francis Crick considers them the "garbage disposal of the mind" and thinks they are helpful only in their ability to clear out useless information.

Dr. Ernest Hartmann of Tufts University in Boston says, "Being able to remember our dreams is not as important as dreaming sleep itself."[6] Some people who claim to never dream actually dream for hours when observed in a sleep laboratory. They simply don't remember their dreams.

If you don't get enough sleep is it helpful to take a nap the next day?

No. You will probably disturb your sleep that night by taking a nap after a short night's sleep. Scientists recommend "prophylactic napping"—taking a nap *before* a short night's sleep to keep your body well rested and on schedule.

Sleep Problems

How many people suffer from insomnia?

Doctors estimate that 100 million people suffer from transient insomnia—the short term inability to sleep. About 20 million people struggle with chronic insomnia, and about 70 percent of them seek medical help.

What is the most common cause of insomnia?

Psychological or psychiatric problems, such as depression.

How do you know if snoring is a sign of a sleep disorder?

You can't know for sure without consulting a doctor, but if you seem to sleep poorly, snore regularly, and if your snoring sometimes sounds like gasping (you can tape-record it), you should consult a physician. Sleep apnea, of which these are symptoms, is most often found in people who are overweight and over the age of 50.

What is sleeping sickness?

Some people confuse narcolepsy, the tendency to fall asleep at inappropriate times, with sleeping sickness, which is a parasitic infection transmitted by bugs and found most often in Africa.

Sleep and Age

Is it important for children to sleep a certain amount of time?

Children have different needs for sleep, just as adults do, but it is more important for children to sleep because they are physically growing and many growth hormones are more concentrated during sleeping hours. Children also are learning much about their environment, which is aided by REM sleep.

Do older people need less sleep?

There are different theories on this. Some doctors believe that older people need less sleep. Others feel that we sleep less efficiently as we age and need as much sleep yet still feel less rested.

Is narcolepsy a disease? Is it contagious?

No. Narcolepsy is an inherited sleep disorder. Scientists have been able to identify the chromosome that carries the gene causing narcolepsy. Drug therapy is sometimes, but not always, successful in treating this condition.

For more information on sleep disorders, read *Overcoming Insomnia* by Dr. Donald Sweeney or *Insomnia and Other Sleeping Problems* by Peter Lambley.

Appendix 1

Sleep Clinics

Introduction

Sleep disorders include problems with sleeping, staying awake, and troublesome behavior during sleep.

The American Sleep Disorders Association is dedicated to maintaining high medical standards in the diagnosis and treatment of these difficulties.

The ASDA has two membership branches: Center/Laboratory Members and Individual Members. This is a roster of Accredited Member Centers that provide the diagnosis and treatment of all types of sleep related disorders, and Accredited Member Specialty Laboratories that specialize only in sleep-related breathing disorders.

Interested parties should consult the nearest facility for more information on specific sleep problems and for appointments.

Alabama

Sleep Disorders Center of Alabama
Affiliated with Baptist Medical Center Montclair
800 Montclair Road
Birmingham, AL 35213
Attn: Vernon Pegram, Ph.D., A.C.P.
205-592-5650

Sleep-Wake Disorders Center
University of Alabama
University Station
Birmingham, AL 35294
Attn: Virgil Wooten, M.D., A.C.P.
205-934-7110

Sleep Disorders Laboratory
The Children's Hospital of Alabama*
1600 7th Avenue South
Birmingham, AL 35233
Attn: Raymond K. Lyrene, M.D.
205-939-9386

Sleep Disorders Center of Huntsville Hospital
Huntsville Hospital
101 Sivley Road
Huntsville, AL 35801
Attn: Paul LeGrand, M.D., A.C.P.;
Debra J. Collier, R.R.T., R.PSG.T.
205-533-8553

Sleep Disorders Center
Mobile Infirmary Medical Center
P.O. Box 2144
Mobile, AL 36652
Attn: Robert P. Dawkins, Ph.D., A.C.P.
205-431-5559

Alaska

No Accredited Members

---

* Accredited Specialty Laboratory for Sleep-Related Breathing Disorders

Arizona

Sleep Disorders Center
Good Samaritan Medical Center
1111 East McDowell Road
Phoenix, AZ 85006
Attn: Richard M. Riedy, M.D., A.C.P.
602-239-5815

Sleep Disorders Center
Humana Hospital–Desert Valley
3929 East Bell Road
Phoenix, AZ 85032
Attn: Jeffrey S. Gitt, D.O., A.C.P.; Tim
   Schwaiger, M.A.
602-867-5686

Sleep Disorders Center
University of Arizona
1501 North Campbell Avenue
Tucson, AZ 85724
Attn: Stuart F. Quan, M.D., A.C.P.
602-694-6112

Arkansas

Sleep Disorders Center
Arkansas Children's Hospital
800 Marshall Street
Little Rock, AR 72202-3591
Attn: Debra H. Fiser, M.D.
501-370-1893

**Sleep Disorders Diagnostic & Research
   Center**
University of Arkansas for Medical
   Sciences
4301 West Markham, Slot 594
Little Rock, AR 72205
Attn: Lawrence Scrima, Ph.D., A.C.P.;
   F. Charles Hiller, M.D.
501-686-6300

Sleep Disorders Center
Baptist Medical Center
9601 I-630, Exit 7
Little Rock, AR 72205-7299
Attn: Robert C. Galbraith, M.D., A.C.P.;
   James Phillips, M.D.
501-227-1902

California

WMCA Sleep Disorder Center
Western Medical Center–Anaheim
1101 South Anaheim Boulevard
Anaheim, CA 92805
Attn: Louis McNabb, M.D., A.C.P.
714-491-1159

Sleep Disorders Center
Downey Community Hospital
11500 Brookshire Avenue
Downey, CA 90241
Attn: Mark J. Buchfuhrer, M.D., A.C.P.
213-806-5280

Sleep Disorders Institute
St. Jude Hospital and
   Rehabilitation Center
101 East Valencia Mesa Drive
Fullerton, CA 92634
Attn: Robert Roethe, M.D.; Justine A.
   Petrie, M.D.; Steven Waldman, M.D.
714-871-3280

Sleep Disorders Center
Scripps Clinic Research
   Foundation
10666 North Torrey Pines Road
La Jolla, CA 92037
Attn: Milton Erman, M.D., A.C.P.
619-554-8087

Sleep Disorders Center
Grossmont District Hospital
P.O. Box 158
5555 Grossmont Center Drive
La Mesa, CA 92044-0300
Attn: Larry N. Ayers, M.D., A.C.P.;
   Linda Neu Ollis
619-589-4488

Respiratory Sleep Laboratory
Antelope Valley Hospital Medical
   Center*
1600 West Avenue J
Lancaster, CA 93534
Attn: Pradeep B. Damie, M.D.; Hal
   Chestnut, Director of Therapies
805-949-5000

The Sleep Disorders Center
The Hospital of the Good
  Samaritan
616 South Witmer Street
Los Angeles, CA 90017
Attn: F. Grant Buckle, M.D., F.C.C.P.,
  A.C.P.; Beverly Martin, R-CPT
213-977-2206

UCLA Sleep Disorders Clinic
Department of Neurology
Room 1184, RNRC
710 Westwood Plaza
Los Angeles, CA 90024
Attn: Donna Arand, Ph.D., A.C.P.
213-206-8005

North Valley Sleep Disorders Center
11550 Indian Hills Road,
  Suite 291
Mission Hills, CA 91345
Attn: Elliott R. Phillips, M.D., A.C.P.;
  Michael M. Stevenson, Ph.D., A.C.P.
818-361-0996

Sleep Disorders Center
Hoag Memorial Hospital
  Presbyterian
301 Newport Boulevard
Newport Beach, CA 92663
Attn: Paul A. Selecky, M.D., A.C.P.
714-760-2070

Sleep Apnea Center
Merritt-Peralta Medical Center*
450 30th Street
Oakland, CA 94609
Attn: Jerrold A. Kram, M.D., A.C.P.;
  Richard A. Nusser, M.D., A.C.P.
415-451-4900, x2273

Sleep Disorders Center
University of California Irvine Medical
  Center
101 City Drive South
Orange, CA 92668
Attn: Sarah S. Mosko, Ph.D., A.C.P.;
  Robert A. Moore, M.D., A.C.P.
714-634-5105

Sleep Disorders Center
Huntington Memorial Center*
100 Congress Street
Pasadena, CA 91105
Attn: Robert S. Eisenberg, M.D., F.A.C.P.
818-397-3061

Sleep Disorders Center
Pomona Valley Hospital
  Medical Center
1798 North Garey Avenue
Pomona, CA 91767
Attn: Dennis Nicholson, M.D., A.C.P.;
  Bhupat Desai, M.D.; Melvin Butler,
  M.D.; Michael H. Bonnet, M.D.,
  A.C.P.
714-865-9135

Sleep Disorders Center
Sequoia Hospital
Whipple and Alameda
Redwood City, CA 94062
Attn: Bernhard Votteri, M.D., A.C.P.;
  Robert N. Pavy, M.D.
415-367-5137

Sutter Sleep Disorders Laboratory
Sutter Hospitals*
52nd and F Streets
Sacramento, CA 95819
Attn: Donald E. Paulson
916-733-1070

**San Diego Regional Sleep
  Disorders Center**
Harbor View Medical Center and
  Hospital
120 Elm Street
San Diego, CA 92101
Attn: Renata Shafor, M.D., A.C.P.
619-235-3176

Sleep Disorders Center
Pacific Presbyterian
  Medical Center
P.O. Box 7999
San Francisco, CA 94120
Attn: Jon F. Sassin, M.D., A.C.P.;
  Bruce T. Adornato, M.D., F.A.C.P.
415-923-3336

Sleep Disorders Clinic
Stanford University Medical Center
211 Quarry Road, N2A
Stanford, CA 94305
Attn: Christian Guilleminault, M.D.,
  A.C.P.
415-723-6601

Southern California Sleep Apnea Center
Lombard Medical Group*
2230 Lynn Road
Thousand Oaks, CA 91360
Attn: Ronald A. Popper, M.D.
805-495-1066

Sleep Disorders Center
Torrance Memorial Hospital
3330 Lomita Boulevard
Torrance, CA 90509
Attn: Lawrence W. Kneisley, M.D., A.C.P.
213-517-4617

Sleep Disorders Center
Kaweah Delta District Hospital*
400 West Mineral King Avenue
Visalia, CA 93291
Attn: William Winn, M.D.
209-625-7303

Pediatric Sleep Apnea Laboratory
Queen of the Valley Hospital*
1115 South Sunset Avenue
West Covina, CA 91790
Attn: Gilbert I. Martin, M.D.; Bruce D. Sindel, M.D.
818-962-4011

Colorado

Sleep Disorders Center
University of Colorado Health Sciences Center
700 Delaware Street
Denver, CO 80204
Attn: Martin L. Reite, M.D., A.C.P.
303-592-7278

Cardio-Respiratory Sleep Disorders Center
National Jewish Center for Immunology and Respiratory Medicine*
1400 Jackson
Denver, CO 80206
Attn: Richard J. Martin, M.D.
303-398-1426

Connecticut

New Haven Sleep Disorders Center
100 York Street
University Towers
New Haven, CT 06511
Attn: Robert K. Watson, Ph.D., A.C.P.; Ian Sholomskas, M.D.
203-776-9578

Delaware

No Accredited Members

District of Columbia

Sleep Disorders Center
Georgetown University Hospital
3800 Reservoir Road, Northwest
Washington, DC 20007-2197
Attn: Samuel J. Potolicchio, Jr., M.D., A.C.P.
202-784-3610

Florida

Sleep Disorder Laboratory
Broward General Medical Center*
Pulmonary Department
1600 South Andrews Avenue
Fort Lauderdale, FL 33316
Attn: Glenn R. Singer, M.D.
305-355-5534

Sleep-Related Breathing Disorders Center
Baptist Medical Center*
800 Prudential Drive
Jacksonville, FL 32207
Attn: Laurence A. Smolley, M.D., A.C.P.
904-393-2909

Center for Sleep Disordered Breathing*
P.O. Box 2982
Jacksonville, FL 32203
Attn: William M. Mentz, M.D.
904-387-7300, x8743

Sleep Disorders Center
Mt. Sinai Medical Center
4300 Alton Road
Miami Beach, FL 33140
Attn: Alejandro D. Chediak, M.D.
305-674-2613

Georgia

Sleep Disorders Center
Northside Hospital
1000 Johnson Ferry Road
Atlanta, GA 30342
Attn: James J. Wellman, M.D., A.C.P.;
   D. Alan Lankford, Ph.D., A.C.P.
404-851-8135

Savannah Sleep Disorders Center
Saint Joseph's Hospital
11705 Mercy Boulevard
P.O. Box 60129
Savannah, GA 31420-0129
Attn: Anthony M. Costrini, M.D.; Joel A.
   Greenberg, M.D., A.C.P.
912-927-5141

Hawaii

Sleep Disorders Center of the Pacific
Straub Clinic & Hospital
888 South King Street
Honolulu, HI 96813
Attn: James W. Pearce, M.D., A.C.P.
808-522-4448

Idaho

No Accredited Members

Illinois

Sleep Disorders Center
Rush–Presbyterian–St. Luke's
1753 West Congress Parkway
Chicago, IL 60612
Attn: Rosalind Cartwright, Ph.D., A.C.P.
312-942-5440

Sleep Disorders Center
University Chicago
5841 South Maryland, Box 425
Chicago, IL 60637
Attn: Jean-Paul Spire, M.D., A.C.P.
312-702-0648

**Center for Sleep-Related Breathing
   Disorders**
Decatur Memorial Hospital*
2300 North Edward
Decatur, IL 62526
Attn: Michael J. Zia, M.D.
217-877-8121, x5405

Sleep Disorders Center
Evanston Hospital
2650 Ridge Avenue
Evanston, IL 60201
Attn: Richard S. Rosenberg, Ph.D.,
   A.C.P.
708-570-2567

**C. Duane Morgan Sleep Disorders
   Center**
Methodist Medical Center of Illinois
221 Northeast Glen Oak
Peoria, IL 61636
Attn: Arthur Fox, M.D., A.C.P.
309-672-4966

Carle Regional Sleep Disorders Center
602 West University
Urbana, IL 61801
Attn: Daniel Picchietti, M.D., A.C.P.;
   Donald A. Greeley, M.D.
217-337-3364

Indiana

Sleep/Wake Disorders Center
Community Hospitals of Indianapolis
1500 North Ritter Avenue
Indianapolis, IN 46219
Attn: Marvin E. Vollmer, M.D., A.C.P.
317-353-4275

Sleep Disorders Center
Winona Memorial Hospital
3232 North Meridian Street
Indianapolis, IN 46208
Attn: Kenneth N. Wiesert, M.D., A.C.P.
317-927-2100

Sleep Alertness Center
Lafayette Home Hospital
2400 South Street
Lafayette, IN 47903
Attn: Fredrick C. Robinson, M.D., A.C.P.
317-447-6811

Iowa

Sleep Disorders Center
Mercy Hospital*
West Central Park at Marquette
Davenport, IA 52804
Attn: Michael H. Laws, M.D.
319-383-1071

St. Luke's Sleep Disorders Center For Sleep-Related Breathing Disorders*
1227 East Rusholme Street
Davenport, IA 52803
Attn: Akshay Mahadevia, M.D.
319-326-6740

Sleep Disorders Center
Iowa Methodist Medical Center
1200 Pleasant Street
Des Moines, IA 50309
Attn: Randall R. Hanson, M.D.
515-283-5094

Kansas

No Accredited Members

Kentucky

Sleep Disorders Center
St. Joseph's Hospital
One St. Joseph Drive
Lexington, KY 40504
Attn: Robert P. Granacher, Jr., M.D., A.C.P.
606-278-0444

Sleep Apnea Laboratory
University of Kentucky College of Medicine*
MN 578, Department of Medicine
800 Rose Street
Lexington, KY 40536-0084
Attn: Barbara Phillips, M.D.
606-233-5290

Sleep Disorders Center
Humana Hospital–Audobon
One Audobon Plaza Drive
Louisville, KY 40217
Attn: David H. Winslow, M.D., A.C.P.

Louisana

Tulane Sleep Disorders Center
1415 Tulane Avenue
New Orleans, LA 70112
Attn: Gregory S. Ferriss, M.D., A.C.P.
504-584-3592

LSU Sleep Disorders Center
Louisana State University Medical Center
P.O. Box 33932
Shreveport, LA 71130-3932
Attn: Andrew L. Chesson, Jr., M.D., A.C.P.
318-674-5365

Maine

Sleep Laboratory
Maine Medical Center*
22 Bramhall Street
Portland, ME 04102
Attn: George E. Bokinsky, Jr., M.D.
207-871-2279

Maryland

The Johns Hopkins Sleep Disorders Center
Hopkins Bayview Research Campus
Francis Scott Key Medical Center
301 Bayview Boulevard
Baltimore, MD 21224
Attn: Philip L. Smith, M.D.
301-550-0571

The Maryland Sleep Diagnostic Center
Ruxton Towers, Suite 211
8415 Bellona Lane
Baltimore, MD 21204
Attn: Thomas E. Hobbins, M.D.;
Cartan B. Kraft, M.B.A.
301-494-9773

National Capitol Sleep Center
4520 East West Highway, Number 406
Bethesda, MD 20814
Attn: Robert Lewit, M.D.
301-656-9515

Massachusetts

Sleep Disorders Unit
Beth Israel Hospital
330 Brookline Avenue, KS430
Boston, MA 02215
Attn: Jean K. Matheson, M.D., A.C.P.;
J. Woodrow Weiss, M.D., A.C.P.
617-735-3237

Michigan

Sleep/Wake Disorders Unit (127B)
VA Medical Center
Southfield & Outer Drive
Allen Park, MI 48101
Attn: Sheldon Kapen, M.D., A.C.P.
313- 562-6000, x3662

Sleep Disorders Center
University of Michigan Hospitals
1500 East Medical Center Drive
Med Inn C433, Box 0842
Ann Arbor, MI 48109-0115
Attn: Michael S. Aldrich, M.D., A.C.P.
313-936-9068

Sleep Disorders Center
Henry Ford Hospital
2799 West Grand Boulevard
Detroit, MI 48202
Attn: Frank Zorick, M.D., A.C.P.
313-972-1800

Sleep Disorders Program
Ingham Medical Center
2025 South Washington Avenue,
  Suite 300
Lansing, MI 48910-0817
Attn: Paul Gouin, M.D., A.C.P.
517-334-2510

Sleep Disorders Institute
44199 Dequindre, Suite 403
Troy, MI 48098
Attn: Rahul Sangal, M.D., A.C.P.
313-54-SLEEP

Minnesota

**Duluth Regional Sleep Disorders
  Center**
St. Mary's Medical Center
407 East Third Street
Duluth, MN 55805
Attn: Peter K. Franklin, M.D.
218-726-4692

Sleep Disorders Center
Abbott Northwestern Hospital
800 East 28th Street at Chicago Avenue
Minneapolis, MN 55407
Attn: Wilfred A. Corson, M.D., A.C.P.
612-863-3200

**Minnesota Regional Sleep Disorders
  Center #860**
Hennepin County Medical Center
701 Park Avenue South
Minneapolis, MN 55415
Attn: Mark Mahowald, M.D., A.C.P.
612-347-6288

Sleep Disorders Center
Mayo Clinic
200 First Street, Southwest
Rochester, MN 55905
Attn: Peter J. Hauri, Ph.D., A.C.P.;
  John W. Shepard, Jr., M.D., A.C.P.
507-286-8900

Sleep Disorders Center
Methodist Hospital
6500 Excelsior Boulevard
St. Louis Park, MN 55426
Attn: Ted Berman, M.D., A.C.P.
612-932-6083

Mississippi

Sleep Disorders Center
Memorial Hospital at Gulfport
P.O. Box 1810
Gulfport, MS 39501
Attn: Joe A. Jackson, M.D., A.C.P.
601-865-3152 or 865-3495

Sleep Disorders Center
University of Mississippi Medical
  Center
2500 North State Street
Jackson, MS 39216-4505
Attn: Lawrence S. Schoen, Ph.D., A.C.P.
601-984-4820

Missouri

Sleep Disorders Center
Research Medical Center
2316 East Meyer Boulevard
Kansas City, MO 64132-1199
Attn: Jon D. Magee, Ph.D.
816-276-4222

Sleep Disorders and Research Center
Deaconess Hospital
6150 Oakland Avenue
St. Louis, MO 63139
Attn: James K. Walsh, Ph.D., A.C.P.
314-768-3100

Sleep Disorders Center
St. Louis University Medical Center
1221 South Grand Boulevard
St. Louis, MO 63104
Attn: Kristyna M. Hartse, Ph.D., A.C.P.
314-577-8705

Sleep Disorders Center
L.E. Cox Medical Center
3801 South National Avenue
Springfield, MO 65807
Attn: Edward Gwin, M.D.
417-885-6189

Montana

No Accredited Members

Nebraska

Sleep Disorders Center
Lutheran Medical Center*
515 South 26th Street
Omaha, NE 68103
Attn: Robert Ellingson, Ph.D., M.D.;
    John D. Roehrs, M.D.
402-536-6784

Nevada

No Accredited Members

New Hampshire

Sleep-Wake Disorders Center
Hampstead Hospital
East Road
Hampstead, NH 03841
Attn: J. Gila Lindsley, Ph.D., A.C.P.;
    R. James Farrer, M.D.
603-329-5311, x240

Dartmouth-Hitchcock Sleep Disorders Center
Department of Psychiatry
Dartmouth Medical School
Hanover, NH 03756
Attn: Michael Sateia, M.D., A.C.P.
603-646-7534

New Jersey

Sleep Disorders Center
Newark Beth Israel Medical Center
201 Lyons Avenue
Newark, NJ 07112
Attn: Monroe S. Karetzky, M.D.
201-926-7163

New Mexico

No Accredited Members

New York

Sleep-Wake Disorders Center
Montefiore Hospital
111 East 210th Street
Bronx, NY 10467
Attn: Michael J. Thorpy, M.D., A.C.P.
212-920-4841

Sleep Disorders Center of Western New York
Millard Fillmore Hospital
3 Gates Circle
Buffalo, NY 14209
Attn: Edwin J. Manning, M.D.;
    Andras J. Vari, M.D.
716-887-4776

Sleep Disorders Center
Columbia-Presbyterian Medical Center
161 Fort Washington Avenue
New York, NY 10032
    -or-
38 East 61st Street
New York, NY 10021
Attn: Neil B. Kavey, M.D., A.C.P.
212-305-1860

Sleep Disorders Center of Rochester
2110 Clinton Avenue South
Rochester, NY 14618
Attn: Donald W. Greenblatt, M.D., A.C.P.
716-442-4141

Sleep Disorders Center
University Hospital
MR 120 A
Stony Brook, NY 11794-7139
Attn: Wallace B. Mendelson, M.D., A.C.P.
516-444-2916

The Sleep Center
Community General Hospital
Broad Road
Syracuse, NY 13215
Attn: Robert E. Westlake, M.D.; James T.
    Moore, R.PSG.T
315-492-5877

The Sleep Laboratory
St. Joseph's Hospital Health Center
301 Prospect Avenue
Syracuse, NY 13203
Attn: Edward T. Downing, M.D.,
    F.C.C.P.; Frank L. Smith
315-448-5870

Sleep-Wake Disorders Center
New York Hospital–Cornell Medical
    Center
21 Bloomingdale Road
White Plains, NY 10605
Attn: Charles Pollak, M.D., A.C.P.
914-997-5751

North Carolina

Sleep Disorders Center
University Memorial Hospital
P.O. Box 560727
W.T. Harris Boulevard at US 29
Charlotte, NC 28256
Attn: Dennis L. Hill, M.D., A.C.P.
704-547-9556

North Dakota

Sleep Disorders Center
St. Luke's Hospital
720 4th Street North
Fargo, ND 58122
Attn: Joseph M. Cullen, M.D., A.C.P.
701-234-5673

Ohio

Sleep Disorders Center
Bethesda Oak Hospital
619 Oak Street
Cincinnati, OH 45206
Attn: Milton Kramer, M.D., A.C.P.
513-569-6320

The Center for Research in Sleep
    Disorders
Affiliated with Mercy Hospital of
    Hamilton/Fairfield
1275 East Kemper Road
Cincinnati, OH 45246
Attn: Martin B. Scharf, Ph.D., A.C.P.
513-671-3101

Sleep Disorders Center
The Cleveland Clinic
    Foundation
9500 Euclid Avenue S53
Cleveland, OH 44195
Attn: Dudley S. Dinner, M.D., A.C.P.
216-444-2165

The Ohio State University Sleep
    Disorders Treatment and Research
    Center
473 West 12th Avenue
Columbus, OH 43210
Attn: Helmut S. Schmidt, M.D., A.C.P.
614-293-8296

The Center for Sleep and Wake
    Disorders
Miami Valley Hospital
Thirty Apple Street, Suite G200
Dayton, OH 45409
Attn: James P. Graham, M.D., A.C.P.
513-220-2515

Sleep Disorders Center
Kettering Medical Center
3535 Southern Boulevard
Kettering, OH 45429-1295
Attn: George G. Burton, M.D.; Lenora
    Gray, M.D.; Massimo DeMarchis,
    Psy.D., A.C.P.
513-296-7805

Sleep Disorders Center
St. Vincent Medical Center
2213 Cherry Street
Toledo, OH 43608-2691
Attn: Joseph I. Shaffer, Ph.D., A.C.P.
419-321-4980

**Northwest Ohio Sleep Disorders
Center**
The Toledo Hospital
2142 North Cove Boulevard
Toledo, OH 43606
Attn: Frank O. Horton III, M.D., A.C.P.
419-471-5629

Oklahoma

No Accredited Members

Oregon

Sleep Disorders Center
Rogue Valley Medical Center
2825 Barnett Road
Medford, OR 97504
Attn: Eric S. Overland, M.D., A.C.P.
503-770-4320

**Pacific Northwest Sleep Disorders
Program**
Good Samaritan Hospital
1130 Northwest 22nd Avenue, Suite 240
Portland, OR 97210
Attn: Gerald B. Rich, M.D., A.C.P.
503-229-8311

Pennsylvania

Sleep Disorders Center
Mercy Hospital of Johnstown
1127 Franklin Street
Johnstown, PA 15905
Attn: Richard Parcinski, D.O., A.C.P.
814-533-1661

Sleep Disorders Center
Jefferson Medical College
1015 Walnut Street, Third Floor
Philadelphia, PA 19107
Attn: Karl Doghramji, M.D., A.C.P.
215-955-6175

Sleep Disorders Center
Department of Neurology
The Medical College of Pennsylvania
3200 Henry Avenue
Philadelphia, PA 19129
Attn: June M. Fry, M.D., Ph.D., A.C.P.
215-842-4250

Sleep Evaluation Center
Western Psychiatric Institute and Clinic
3811 O'Hara Street
Pittsburgh, PA 15213-2593
Attn: Charles F. Reynolds III, M.D.,
A.C.P.
412-624-2246

Sleep Disorders Center
Department of Neurology
Crozer-Chester Medical Center
Upland-Chester, PA 19013
Attn: Calvin R. Stafford, M.D., A.C.P.
215-447-2689

Rhode Island

Sleep Apnea Laboratory
Rhode Island Hospital*
593 Eddy Street, APC 479-A
Providence, RI 02903
Attn: Richard P. Millman, M.D., A.C.P.;
Elizabeth Simas
401-277-5306

South Carolina

**Sleep Disorders Center of South
Carolina**
Baptist Medical Center
Taylor at Marion Streets
Columbia, SC 29220
Attn: Richard Bogan, M.D., F.C.C.P.,
A.C.P.; Sharon S. Ellis, M.D.
803-771-5847

**Sleep Disorders Center of the
Greenville Hospital System**
Greenville Memorial Hospital
701 Grove Road
Greenville, SC 29605
Attn: Freddie E. Wilson, M.D., A.C.P.;
Joe W. Pollard, Jr.
803-242-8916

Children's Sleep Disorders Center
Self Memorial Hospital*
1325 Spring Street
Greenwood, SC 29646
Attn: Terry A. Marshall, M.D.
803-227-4449 or 227-4206

Sleep Disorders Center
Spartanburg Regional Medical Center
101 East Wood Street
Spartanburg, SC 29303
Attn: Wilson P. Smith, Jr., M.D., A.C.P.
803-591-6524

South Dakota

The Sleep Center
Rapid City Regional Hospital
353 Fairmont Boulevard
P.O. Box 6000
Rapid City, SD 57709
Attn: K. Alan Kelts, M.D., A.C.P.
605-341-7378

Sleep Disorders Center
Sioux Valley Hospital
1100 South Euclid
Sioux Falls, SD 57117-5039
Attn: Richard D. Hardie, M.D., A.C.P.;
Brian Hurley, M.D., A.C.P.
605-333-6302

Tennessee

Sleep Disorders Center
Ft. Sanders Regional Medical Center
1901 West Clinch Avenue
Knoxville, TN 37916
Attn: Thomas G. Higgins, M.D., A.C.P.;
Bert A. Hampton, M.D., A.C.P.
615-541-1375

Sleep Disorders Center
St. Mary's Medical Center
Oak Hill Avenue
Knoxville, TN 37917
Attn: Russell Rosenberg, Ph.D., A.C.P.
615-971-7529

BMH Sleep Disorders Center
Baptist Memorial Hospital
899 Madison Avenue
Memphis, TN 38146
Attn: Helio Lemmi, M.D., A.C.P.
901-522-5704

Sleep Disorders Center
Saint Thomas Hospital
P.O. Box 380
Nashville, TN 37202
Attn: J. Brevard Haynes, Jr., M.D.,
A.C.P.
615-386-2068

**West Side Hospital Sleep
Disorders Center**
West Side Hospital
2221 Murphy Avenue
Nashville, TN 37203
Attn: David A. Jarvis, M.D.; J. Michael
Bolds, M.D., A.C.P.
615-329-6292

Texas

Sleep-Wake Disorders Center
Presbyterian Hospital
8200 Walnut Hill Lane
Dallas, TX 75231
Attn: Philip M. Becker, M.D., A.C.P.
214-696-8563

Sleep/Wake Disorders Center
RHD Memorial Medical Center
P.O. Box 819094
LBJ Freeway at Webbs Chapel
Dallas, TX 75381-9094
Attn: James P. Loftin, M.D., A.C.P.;
Robert S. Obregon, R.PSG.T
214-888-7079

Sleep Disorders Center
Sun Towers Hospital
1801 North Oregon
El Paso, TX 79902
Attn: Gonzalo Diaz, M.D.
915-532-6281

**All Saints Sleep Disorders Diagnostic
and Treatment Center**
All Saints Episcopal Hospital
1400 8th Avenue
Fort Worth, TX 76104
Attn: Edgar Lucas, Ph.D., A.C.P.
817-927-6120

Sleep Disorders Center
Department of Psychiatry
Baylor College of Medicine and VA
Medical Center
Houston, TX 77030
Attn: Ismet Karacan, M.D., A.C.P.
713-799-4886

Sleep Disorders Center
Sam Houston Memorial Hospital
8300 Waterbury, Suite 350
Houston, TX 77055
Attn: Todd J. Swick, M.D.; Andrea K.
Zebrak, B.S., R.PSG.T
713-973-6483

Sleep Disorders Center
Scott and White Clinic
2401 South 31st Street
Temple, TX 76508
Attn: Francisco Perez-Guerra, M.D.,
  A.C.P.
817-774-2554

Utah

Sleep Disorders Center
Utah Neurological Clinic
1055 North 300 West, Suite 400
Provo, UT 84604
Attn: John M. Andrews, M.D., A.C.P.
801-379-7400

Intermountain Sleep Disorders Center
LDS Hospital
325 8th Avenue
Salt Lake City, UT 84143
Attn: James M. Walker, Ph.D., A.C.P.;
  Robert J. Farney, M.D., A.C.P.
801-321-3417

Vermont

No Accredited Members

Virginia

Sleep Disorders Center
Eastern Virginia Medical School
Sentara Norfolk General Hospital
600 Gresham Drive
Norfolk, VA 23507
Attn: Reuben H. McBrayer, M.D.;
  J. Catesby Ware, Ph.D., A.C.P.
804-628-3322

Medical College of Virginia Sleep Disorders Center
Medical College of Virginia
P.O. Box 268–MCV Station
Richmond, VA 23298-0268
Attn: Charles C. Morin, Ph.D.
804-786-1993

Sleep Disorders Center
Community Hospital of Roanoke Valley
P.O. Box 12946
Roanoke, VA 24029
Attn: Thomas W. deBeck, M.D., A.C.P.;
  William S. Elias, M.D., A.C.P.
703-985-8435

Washington

Sleep Disorders Center
Providence Professional Building
Providence Medical Center
550 16th Avenue, Suite 304
Seattle, WA 98124
Attn: Ralph A. Pascualy, M.D., A.C.P.
206-326-5366

Sacred Heart Sleep Apnea Center
Sacred Heart Medical Center*
West 101 Eighth Avenue, TAF-C9
Spokane, WA 99220-4045
Attn: Jeffrey C. Elmer, M.D., A.C.P.;
  Elizabeth Hurd
509-455-4895

West Virginia

No Accredited Members

Wisconsin

Wisconsin Sleep Disorders Center
Gundersen Clinic, Ltd.
1836 South Avenue
La Crosse, WI 54601
Attn: Martin L. Engman, M.D., A.C.P.
608-782-7300

Milwaukee Regional Sleep Disorders Center
Columbia Hospital
2025 East Newport Avenue
Milwaukee, WI 53211
Attn: Marvin R. Wooten, M.D., A.C.P.
414-961-4650

Sleep/Wake Disorders Center
St. Mary's Hospital
2320 North Lake Drive
Milwaukee, WI 53211-4565
Attn: Paul A. Nausieda, M.D.
414-225-8032

Wyoming

No Accredited Members

This list is the Roster of Member Accredited Centers and Laboratories current as of February 28, 1990. For the most current roster please write to the American Sleep Disorders Association, 604 Second Street Southwest, Rochester, MN 55902.

Appendix 2

Where to Find a Light Box

Medic-Light Inc.
Yacht Club Drive
Hopatcong, NJ 07849

The Sun Box Co.
1307 Taft St.
Rockville, MD 20850

Appendix 3

Sunrise, Sunset Times for 2 Latitudes

Date	45° Lat Sunrise/Sunset	35° Lat Sunrise/Sunset
January 1	7:38/4:29	7:08/5:00
January 15	7:35/4:45	7:08/5:12
February 1	7:20/5:07	7:00/5:29
February 15	7:01/5:28	6:46/5:43
March 1	6:38/5:48	6:29/5:56
March 15	6:12/6:06	6:11/6:08
April 1	5:41/6:28	5:47/6:21
April 15	5:15/6:46	5:28/6:33
May 1	4:47/7:06	5:09/6:46
May 15	4:31/7:26	4:56/6:57
June 1	4:16/7:40	4:47/7:09
June 15	4:13/7:49	4:46/7:16
July 1	4:17/7:50	4:50/7:18
July 15	4:28/7:44	4:57/7:14
August 1	4:45/7:27	5:09/7:03
August 15	5:02/7:06	5:20/6:48
September 1	5:22/6:37	5:33/6:27
September 15	5:39/6:11	5:43/6:07
October 1	5:58/5:40	5:55/5:44
October 15	6:16/5:15	6:06/5:25
November 1	6:39/4:48	6:21/5:06
November 15	6:58/4:31	6:35/4:54
December 1	7:18/4:20	6:50/4:48
December 15	7:31/4:19	7:01/4:50

DST* (bracket spanning April 1 through September 15)

*Daylight Savings Time in effect. Move times up by one hour if observed.

Notes

1. The 13-Month Year

1. Project Sleep was conducted by the National Program on Insomnia and Sleep Disorders and administered through the Department of Health and Human Services in 1979. Film and tape materials on sleep apnea, narcolepsy/cataplexy, and nocturnal myoclonus are available upon request through the Association of Sleep Disorders Centers.

2. Ibid., "Insomnia" tape.

3. *USA Today*, n.d. Although Dr. Sack was not the first person to discover the link between sleep and depression, the article quoting him was the first time I became aware of this theory.

   Other researchers have studied the effects of total sleep deprivation, partial sleep deprivation, and REM sleep deprivation on depressives. For a more thorough discussion of the ways sleep may be manipulated to treat depressive patients, see *Human Sleep* by Wallace Mendelson (New York: Plenum Publishing, 1987), 269–94.

4. Dr. Mangalore Pai quoted in Richard Trubo, *How to Get a Good Night's Sleep* (Boston: Little, Brown & Co., 1978), 40.

5. James Horne, *Why We Sleep* (London: Oxford University Press, 1988), 1.

6. Sandy Rovner, "Health," *Washington Post* (April 2, 1988).

7. Study conducted by Dr. Ernest Hartmann, director of the Sleep Laboratory at Boston Hospital, and reported in his book, *The Functions of Sleep* (New Haven: Yale University Press, 1973). (Longer-sleepers were also often found to be very creative.)

2. Sleep 101

1. Horne, 4.

2. Trubo, 44.

3. Horne, 5.

4. Peter Lambley, *Insomnia and Other Sleeping Problems* (New York: Pinnacle Books, 1982), 33.

5. Lambley, 38

6. Dr. Peter Hauri and Dr. Shirley Linde, *No More Sleepless Nights* (New York: John Wiley and Sons, 1990), 9.

7. Trubo, 45.

8. Wilse Webb, *Sleep, the Gentle Tyrant* (New York: Prentice-Hall, 1975), 23.

9. Mattlin, 69.

10. Mattlin, 70.

11. See "What Is Normal Sleep?" in Lynne Lamberg, *The AMA's Guide to Better Sleep* (New York: Random House, 1984), 16.

12. Horne, 5.

13. Richard M. Coleman, *Wide Awake at 3:00 A.M.* (San Francisco: W. H. Freeman, 1986), 71.

14. *U.S. News and World Report* (February 10, 1988): 64.

15. Horne, 13–14.

16. *The New York Times* (September 24, 1987): 1.

17. Everett Mattlin, *Sleep Less, Live More* (New York: J. B. Lippincott, 1979), 62.

18. Horne, 37–42.

19. Horne, 52.

20. Horne, 46.

21. Richard Podell, *Doctor, Why Am I So Tired?* (New York: Fawcett Books, 1987).

22. Donald Sweeney, *Overcoming Insomnia* (New York: G. P. Putnam & Sons, 1980).

23. Podell, 251–58.

24. Wallace Mendelson, *Human Sleep* (New York: Plenum Publishing, 1987), 19.

25. Lamberg, 156.

3. The Great Escape

1. Marc Beauchamp, "Asleep on the Job," *Forbes* (May 30, 1988): 292.

2. Rob Krakovitz, *High Energy* (New York: Ballantine, 1986), 39.

3. Lamberg, 35.

4. Jesse A. Stoff and Charles R. Pellegrino, *Chronic Fatigue Syndrome* (New York: Random House, 1988), 59–79.

5. Peter Whybrow and Robert Bohr, *The Hibernation Response* (New York: Morrow, 1988).

6. Holly Atkinson, *Women and Fatigue* (New York: Pocket Books, 1985), 107.

7. Trubo, 118.

8. Lamberg, 244.

4. Step 1: Self-Assessment

1. Richard M. Coleman, *Wide Awake at 3:00 A.M.* (San Francisco: W. H. Freeman, 1986), 71.

2. Lamberg, 244.

3. Bernie S. Siegel, *Love, Medicine and Miracles* (New York: Harper & Row, 1986), 69.

4. Lamberg, 34.

5. Ellen Goodman, *Close to Home* (New York: Fawcett Crest Books), 111.

7. Step 4: Patterning

1. *Los Angeles Times* (July 27, 1988):1.

8. Step 5: Diet and Exercise

1. Atkinson, 107.

9. Step 6: Efficient Sleep

1. Hauri and Linde, 72.

2. Horne.

10. Questions and Answers

1. Coleman, 19.

2. *Working Woman* (September 1985): 151.

3. *Washington Post* (December 8, 1987): D10.

4. *Discover* (April 1987): 12.

5. *Nation's Business* (December 1987): 72.

6. *Psychology Today* (October 1984): 16.

Selected Bibliography

Anonymous. "How to Get a Good Night's Sleep—Interview with Merrill Mitler," *U.S. News and World Report* (January 10, 1983): 66–69.

Anonymous. "Why You Can't Sleep—Interview with Wallace Mendelson," *U.S. News and World Report* (February 10, 1986): 64–68.

Anonymous. "Sleep Loss Said Not to Hurt Work of Medical Residents," *New York Times* (September 24, 1987): 1.

Associated Press. "FDA Warns on Use of L-Tryptophan," *The Washington Post* (November 12, 1989): A16.

Atkinson, Holly. *Women and Fatigue.* New York: Pocket Books, 1985.

Beauchamp, Marc. "Asleep on the Job," *Forbes* (May 30, 1988): 292.

Begley, Sharon. "The Stuff That Dreams Are Made Of," *Newsweek* (August 14, 1989): 40–47.

Benson, Herbert. *Your Maximum Mind.* New York: Random House, 1987.

Bolles, Richard Nelson. *What Color Is Your Parachute?* Berkeley: Ten Speed Press, 1984.

Borbely, Alexander. *Secrets of Sleep.* New York: Basic Books, 1986.

Byrd, Robert. "L-Tryptophan Pills Cause Blood Illness," *The Orange County Register* (November 25, 1989): A1.

Carnegie, Dale. *How to Stop Worrying and Start Living.* New York: Simon and Schuster, 1975.

Coleman, Richard. *Wide Awake at 3:00 A.M.* New York: W. H. Freeman, 1986.

Cooper, Kenneth. *Aerobics.* New York: Bantam, 1975.

Delaney, Gayle. *Living Your Dreams.* New York: Harper & Row, 1981.

Ferber, Richard. *Solve Your Child's Sleep Problems.* New York: Simon and Schuster, 1985.

Fisher, Greg et al. *Chronic Fatigue Syndrome.* New York: Warner, 1987.

Franklin, Benjamin. *The Autobiography and Other Writings.* New York: Signet, 1961.

Gardner, David C., and Grace Joely Beatty. *Never Be Tired Again!* New York: Macmillan, 1988.

Hauri, Peter, and Shirley Linde. *No More Sleepless Nights.* New York: John Wiley and Sons, 1990.

Horne, James. *Why We Sleep.* London: Oxford University Press, 1988.

Ingher, Dina. "Is Sleep a Waste of Time?" *Science Digest* (April 1984): 83.

Krakovitz, Rob. *High Energy.* New York: Ballantine, 1986.

LaBerge, Stephen. *Lucid Dreaming.* New York: Ballantine, 1986.

Lamberg, Lynne. *American Medical Association's Guide to Better Sleep.* New York: Random House, 1984.

Lambley, Peter. *Insomnia and Other Sleep Problems.* New York: Windsor Publishing, 1982.

Lavie, Peretz and Shulamist Segal. "Twenty-Four Hour Structure of Sleepiness in Morning and Evening Persons Investigated by Ultrashort Wake Cycles," *Sleep* 12:6 (1989): 522–36.

MacDonald, Gordon. *Ordering Your Private World.* Nashville: Thomas Nelson, 1985.

Mattlin, Everett. *Sleep Less, Live More.* New York: J. B. Lippincott, 1979.

Mendelson, Wallace. *Human Sleep: Research and Clinical Care*. New York: Plenum Publishing Corporation, 1987.

Miller, Laurence. "REM Sleep: Pilot Light of the Mind?" *Psychology Today* (September 1987): 8.

Minirth, Frank et al. *Sweet Dreams*. Grand Rapids: Baker Book House, 1985.

Mirkin, Gabe. "Rise and Shine," *Health* (May 1985): 8.

Peale, Norman Vincent. *The Power of Positive Thinking*. New York: Prentice-Hall, 1956.

Podell, Richard. *Doctor, Why Am I So Tired?* New York: Ballantine, 1987.

Regestein, Quentin. *Sound Sleep*. New York: Simon and Schuster, 1980.

Richards, David. "Wired—One Man's Search for a Good Night's Sleep," *The Washington Post Magazine* (March 25, 1990): 22–25.

Scott, Dru. *How to Put More Time in Your Life*. New York: Rawson, Wade, 1980.

Sher, Barbara. *Wishcraft*. New York: Viking Press, 1979.

Siegel, Bernie. *Love, Medicine, and Miracles*. New York: Harper & Row, 1986.

Siwolop, Sara. "Helping Workers Stay Awake at the Switch," *Business Week* (December 8, 1986): 108.

Snyderman, Nancy. "The Anatomy of Sleep." *ABC Good Morning America* (November 8, 1989).

Soth, Connie. *Insomnia—God's Night School*. Old Tappan, NJ: Revell, 1989.

Standberg, Kjell. Bjorn Beerman, and Gudman Lonnerholm. "Treatment of Sleep Disorders," *National Board of Health and Welfare Drug Information Committee, Sweden* (1984): 183–92.

Stoff, Jesse, and Charles Pellegrino. *Chronic Fatigue Syndrome*. New York: Random House, 1988.

Sweeney, Donald. *Overcoming Insomnia*. New York: Putnam, 1989.

Tec, Leon, *Targets*. New York: Harper & Row, 1980.

Thompson, Larry, and Don Colburn. "Scientists Offer an Explanation for the Monday Morning Blahs," *The Washington Post* (March 24, 1987): A1.

Trubo, Richard. *How to Get a Good Night's Sleep*. Boston: Little, Brown, & Co., 1978.

von Oech, Roger. *A Whack on the Side of the Head*. New York: Warner, 1983.

Whybrow, Peter, and Robert Bohr. *The Hibernation Response*. New York: William Morrow, 1988.